T0282406

The Yale Pharyngeal Residue Severity Rating Scale

Steven B. Leder • Paul D. Neubauer

The Yale Pharyngeal Residue Severity Rating Scale

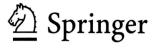 Springer

Steven B. Leder
Department of Surgery
Yale School of Medicine
New Haven, Connecticut
USA

Paul D. Neubauer
Department of Surgery
Yale School of Medicine
New Haven, Connecticut
USA

Additional Material to this book can be downloaded from
http://link.springer.com/book/10.1007/978-3-319-29899-3.

ISBN 978-3-319-29897-9   ISBN 978-3-319-29899-3   (eBook)
DOI 10.1007/978-3-319-29899-3

Library of Congress Control Number: 2016938646

Printed on acid-free paper

This Springer imprint is published by Springer Nature
The registered company is Springer International Publishing AG Switzerland

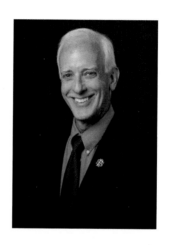

IN MEMORIAM

Steven B. Leder, Ph.D., CCC-SLP

March 22, 1952–May 16, 2016

Dr. Leder will forever be remembered for his dedication to his research and his patients, his kindness, and his sense of humor. His intellect and passion for his work are evident in the pages of this book.

*Severity is in the eye
of the beholder
no longer.*

Preface

We are experienced endoscopists dedicated to providing optimal dysphagia diagnostic and rehabilitative care to our patients. However, we were frustrated that none of the previously published pharyngeal residue severity rating scales met our needs. We knew that pharyngeal residue was a key component of the pharyngeal swallow and that fiberoptic endoscopic evaluation of swallowing (FEES) was the most appropriate instrumental assessment technique to determine pharyngeal residue severity, but we were unable to rate it accurately in our patients, track changes due to therapeutic interventions, or share information with colleagues either across the street or around the world. And research was impossible to do without a reliable and validated pharyngeal severity rating scale. What was needed, we decided, was a pharyngeal residue severity rating scale that was anatomically defined, image-based, reliable, validated, and easy to use.

This was not an easy task. It required reviewing hundreds of archived FEES videos followed by detailed examination of thousands of individual frames prior to selection, analysis, and validation of the final iconic images. As our endoscopist colleagues can appreciate, the images had to be centered and crystal clear, the scope placed at the correct level in the pharynx, all relevant anatomical structures included in the view, and, most importantly, the precise volume of valleculae and pyriform sinus residue corresponding to our severity rating scale had to be depicted. We were able to meet all of these requirements.

You will find our methodology sound, the data supportive, and the recommendations beneficial. We trust that you will incorporate, as we have, the Yale Pharyngeal Residue Severity Rating Scale into your daily clinical practice and that you will find its use helpful to both yourself and your patients. This is reward enough for us.

We have been most gratified with the reception and approval of the Yale Pharyngeal Residue Severity Rating Scale from our colleagues around the world, including speech-language pathologists, otolaryngologists, and other interested deglutologists. We continuously strive to provide state-of-the art patient care and feel enormously privileged to participate in the care of patients to the best of our abilities. And we wish the same for you.

New Haven, CT   Steven B. Leder
                                                 Paul D. Neubauer

Acknowledgments

This book would not have been possible without the support and wisdom of our research co-authors. We gratefully acknowledge the expertise provided by Morton I. Burrell, Douglas J. Van Daele, Denise P. Hersey, and Alfred W. Rademaker. We extend our thanks to our colleagues Catherine M. Camputaro for providing the 3-D images of the pharynx and to Wendell G. Yarbrough for allocating funds for statistical analysis. We must also thank our patients for the privilege of participating in their care as it is for their benefit that the Yale Pharyngeal Residue Severity Rating Scale was developed for both clinical and research uses.

Contents

Chapter 1
Building a Foundation, Defining Terms, and Looking Toward the Future

Introduction

Pharyngeal residue, absence, presence, and severity, has been an integral component of fiberoptic endoscopic evaluation of swallowing (FEES) from the beginning. Why? Because FEES is a uniquely qualified assessment tool to describe the presence of both vallecula and pyriform sinus residue. However, no anatomically defined and image-based pharyngeal residue severity scale existed prior to our work. We will describe the Yale Pharyngeal Residue Severity Rating Scale, a valid, reliable, easy to use, and generalizable tool to rate vallecula and pyriform sinus residue severity patterns. You will be able to understand and use the Yale Pharyngeal Residue Severity Rating Scale for both clinical and scientific research purposes. Clinical uses include accurate classification of vallecula and pyriform sinus residue severity patterns as none, trace, mild, moderate, or severe for diagnostic purposes, determination of functional therapeutic change, and precise dissemination of shared information. Scientific research purposes include tracking outcome measures, demonstrating efficacy of interventions to reduce pharyngeal residue, investigation morbidity and mortality associated with pharyngeal residue severity, and improving training and accuracy of FEES interpretation by students and clinicians alike. We look forward to

S.B. Leder, P.D. Neubauer, *The Yale Pharyngeal Residue Severity Rating Scale*, DOI 10.1007/978-3-319-29899-3_1, © Springer International Publishing Switzerland 2016

you enhancing patient care by adding the Yale Pharyngeal Residue Severity Rating Scale to your clinical toolbox.

It's All About the Bolus

Why write a book about pharyngeal residue? It is simply because pharyngeal residue is a critical component of the pharyngeal phase of swallowing, is a key factor to be identified during fiberoptic endoscopic evaluation of swallowing (FEES), can occur in the vallecula or pyriform sinuses or both, can be predictive of pharyngeal dysphagia and aspiration risk status, can indicate swallowing pathophysiology, and is amenable to therapeutic interventions to promote safer swallowing. It must always be remembered that the difference between a normal and abnormal (hereafter the terms functional and nonfunctional will be used) swallow depends exclusively on the location of the bolus. When the bolus is cleared in either its entirety or when only trace amounts remain in the vallecula and/or pyriform sinuses, the swallow can be considered functional. There is very little risk or consequences of laryngeal penetration and aspiration. But if excess pharyngeal residue remains leading to the probability of increased laryngeal penetration and aspiration risk, then the swallow may be considered nonfunctional. The clinician will attempt some type of therapeutic intervention to reduce residue in the vallecula and pyriform sinuses with the goal of promoting a functional swallow. Therefore, the path the bolus travels defines, for the deglutologist, the severity of the pharyngeal dysphagia, identifies possible pathophysiologic mechanisms, and determines what bolus viscosity and volume modifications and therapeutic interventions may be implemented to promote safe and efficient swallowing.

There are four basic events that comprise the most fundamental findings of a FEES. They are (1) spillage, when the bolus flows into the pharynx before the onset of the reflexive pharyngeal swallow; (2) pharyngeal residue, operationally defined as any part of a bolus that remains in the pharynx, specifically the vallecula and pyriform sinuses, after a swallow has been completed and can vary in volume as evidenced by severity ratings such as trace, mild, moderate, and severe; (3) laryngeal penetration, when the bolus enters the laryngeal vestibule; and (4) aspiration, when the bolus passes below the true vocal folds and into the trachea. This book is focused solely on pharyngeal residue and specifically in the vallecula and pyriform sinuses

The Pharynx

The pharynx is a single tube with a shared pathway for respiration and deglutition. It is positioned caudal to the nasal and oral cavities and cephalic to the larynx and esophagus. The valleculae are located at the junction of the base of the tongue and base of the epiglottis. The pyriform sinuses are positioned inferiorly in the pharynx and on both sides of the larynx. As discussed in detail in Chap. 2, this anatomical position makes the pharynx an integral structure and critically important for a functionally successful swallow.

The Valleculae and Pyriform Sinuses

Pharyngeal residue, operationally defined as pre-swallow secretions and post-swallow food residue in the pharynx not entirely cleared by a swallow, is a clinical predictor of prandial aspiration [1]. An accurate description of pharyngeal residue severity is an important but difficult clinical challenge [2]. Pharyngeal residue occurs in either the valleculae (spaces between the base of the tongue and epiglottis) or the pyriform sinuses (spaces formed on both sides of the pharynx between the fibers of the inferior pharyngeal constrictor muscle and the sides of the thyroid cartilage and lined by orthogonally directed fibers of the palatopharyngeus muscle and pharyngobasilar fascia) [3].

What Can Be Inferred from Pharyngeal Residue?

It is possible, but not always, to determine the pathophysiology of the swallow based upon residue location. The endoscopist should, therefore, always be thinking not only of the severity of

the vallecula and pyriform sinus residue but also why the residue occurred in the first place. The combination of the severity
and pathophysiology can lead to therapeutic interventions that
may prevent residue from occurring or reduce residue severity
enough to promote a functional pharyngeal swallow.

In the majority of cases, vallecula residue occurs due to a
weak pharyngeal swallow characterized by reduced laryngeal
rise resulting in lack of adequate epiglottic inversion, from
reduced base-of-tongue driving force [4, 5], or, most likely, a
combination of these two factors. Also, in the majority of
cases, pyriform sinus residue similarly occurs due to a weak
pharyngeal swallow, but now the consequences are reduced
pharyngeal shortening which prevents the pyriform sinuses
from moving superiorly resulting in retention rather than
emptying of the contents into the now opened upper esophageal sphincter [6]. Additionally, if the upper esophageal
sphincter fails to relax, i.e., due to hypertonicity or spasm, the
bolus cannot pass freely or completely into the esophagus
resulting in pyriform sinus residue and potential spill over
into the airway after the swallow.

Comparison of the Fiberoptic Endoscopic
Evaluation of Swallowing (FEES)
and Videofluoroscopic Swallow Study (VFSS)

Since the time of the first published FEES study [7], pharyngeal residue has been important to identify and treat accord-
ingly. The primary purpose of FEES is to diagnose pharyngeal
phase dysphagia as the superiorly positioned endoscopic
view of the base of the tongue, pharynx, vallecula, larynx, and
pyriform sinuses is unsurpassed by any other imaging technique. Research has shown that pharyngeal and laryngeal
anatomy and physiology as well as residue in the vallecula
and pyriform sinuses pre-swallow, partially peri-swallowing,
and post-swallowing can be determined better with FEES
than with the routine lateral radiographic view provided by

VFSS [8, 9]. Importantly, bolus flow characteristics pre-, peri-, and post-pharyngeal swallowing can be visualized. This permits bolus flow characteristics of fluids of both different viscosities and volumes and different consistencies of foods to be trialed on an individual patient basis for determination of swallow safety [10].

Previously Published Pharyngeal Residue Severity Rating Scales

Different types of scales have attempted to classify pharyngeal residue, but only one has demonstrated the combination of adequate reliability, interpretive validity, and ease of administration to be clinically useful [11]. Scale examples not meeting the criteria for successful clinical use include (1) binary (presence/absence) [5], (2) ordinal (to capture progressively increasing amounts) [1, 12–15], (3) estimation (amount of observed residue as an estimate of the percentage of the original bolus) [9, 16–18], and (4) quantification (computer-based image analysis) [2, 19]. Chapter 3 includes a systematic review of all of the pharyngeal residue rating scales published through 2015. The reader will be able to see the advantages and disadvantages of each scale in order to draw their own conclusions as to the best pharyngeal residue rating scale to use for their own clinical uses and research goals.

It is important to remember that the sole purpose of all of these scales is to rate pharyngeal residue severity. These scales do not determine *why* residue occurs or ascertain the *when* of timing of residue occurrence during swallowing. The only scale, to date, which has provided in vivo, anatomically correct, image-based exemplars of hierarchically organized pharyngeal residue severity ratings against which clinicians can match their clinical judgments of patient swallows is the Yale Pharyngeal Residue Severity Rating Scale [11].

Rationale for the Development of the Yale Pharyngeal Residue Severity Rating Scale

Despite the importance of determining pharyngeal residue severity in the diagnosis of a patient's swallowing abilities when using FEES, only recently has an anatomically defined and image-based pharyngeal residue severity rating scale been developed. In order for any scale to gain widespread acceptance, it must be user friendly, easy to learn, reliable to interpret, and generalizable to all patients undergoing FEES. Such a scale now exists, and it is the Yale Pharyngeal Residue Severity Rating Scale [11].

Deglutologists who use FEES have long lamented the fact that there was no reliable, validated, anatomically defined, image-based, and easily used pharyngeal residue severity rating scale. All that one had to rely on was the "impression" of residue severity, the definition of which varied from endoscopist to endoscopist. This was not an ideal situation. Clinical findings could not be quantified or shared. Efficacy of intervention strategies could not be confirmed. Research could not be defined or replicated. This book is our attempt to address all of these important issues.

When Is It Appropriate to Use the Yale Pharyngeal Residue Severity Rating Scale?

The answer is: *Whenever the clinician wants to determine vallecula and pyriform sinus residue severity.* The Yale Pharyngeal Residue Severity Rating Scale is akin to a ruler. And a ruler can be used whenever the user wishes. The only difference is that the Yale Pharyngeal Residue Severity Rating Scale measures pharyngeal residue, while a ruler measures length. It does not matter *when* the measuring takes place. Expanding on the ruler analogy, when building a table, for example, the carpenter uses the same ruler when first starting, during the building process, and as a final check to make sure all measurements are correct. The ruler can be used as often as needed, and, as the old adage goes, "Measure twice and cut once." In other words, it matters not when the ruler is used, only that a reliable ruler is used for all measurements.

The exact same logic holds true for the Yale Pharyngeal Residue Severity Rating Scale. The scale must come first because what is of prime importance is rating pharyngeal residue in a reliable and validated manner. *Why* residue occurs or *when* the residue occurs is irrelevant to the scale itself. (To reiterate from our example above, *why* the carpenter uses the ruler and *when* the ruler is used is irrelevant to the ruler itself.) Therefore, it is up to the individual clinician to rate pharyngeal residue severity at whatever specific part of the swallow they are interested in. For example, the clinician can determine vallecula and pyriform sinus residue severity immediately after the swallow, 20 s after the swallow, or 1 min after the swallow. It makes no difference because the scale is the measurer that does not vary. The only points of interest after a swallow are determined by the clinician to answer their own specific question.

Sole Purpose of the Yale Pharyngeal Residue Severity Rating Scale

The sole purpose of the Yale Pharyngeal Residue Severity Rating Scale (or for any scale with the goal of determining pharyngeal residue severity) is to allow clinicians and researchers to rate post-swallow vallecula and pyriform sinus residue severity. Consistent with all other pharyngeal residue rating scales [1, 2, 5, 9, 12–19], the Yale Pharyngeal Residue Severity Rating Scale does not determine why residue occurs or ascertain the when of timing of residue occurrence during swallowing. Since all patients present with unique pharyngeal phase swallowing characteristics, it is up to the clinician to determine the *why* and *when* of residue occurrence during swallowing. The superiority of the Yale Pharyngeal Residue Severity Rating Scale is generalizability to all individuals due to its anatomically defined and image-based construction resulting in excellent validity, easy administration, and accurate interpretation by clinicians with a wide range of FEES experience.

Practical Uses of the Yale Pharyngeal Residue Severity Rating Scale

Clinically, the utility, versatility, and efficacy of the Yale Pharyngeal Residue Severity Scale are easily demonstrated. For example, a representative pre-therapy swallow receives a severe vallecula residue severity rating (anatomically defined as the vallecula filled up to the epiglottic rim and with a corresponding image). An intervention strategy, such as effortful swallow or double swallow, is implemented for a set period of time, and a representative post-therapy swallow receives a mild vallecular residue severity rating (anatomically defined as mild pooling with epiglottic ligament visible and with a corresponding image). The clinician can now document efficacy of a specific treatment intervention and either stop, continue, or change strategies. Prior to the development and validation of the Yale Pharyngeal Residue Severity Rating Scale, objective documentation of therapeutic interventions was not possible.

It cannot be stressed enough that the Yale Pharyngeal Residue Rating Scale works well for any swallow, whether it is the first, subsequent clearing, or last swallow. The clinician simply has to match their chosen swallow with its scale mate. In this way, it is possible to determine if, for example, spontaneous or volitional clearing swallows or a throat-clearing maneuver is actually helpful in reducing the amount of residue in the vallecula and pyriform sinuses. Since an important therapeutic goal is to aid pharyngeal clearing [1], this information may result in a functional pharyngeal swallow, can guide intervention strategies, and promote safer swallowing. For example, it is now possible to determine objectively if drinking a small liquid bolus after a puree or solid bolus, an effortful swallow, a double swallow/bolus, a head turn to left or right, and a chin tuck are successful intervention strategies to reduce residue in the vallecula and pyriform sinus.

Versatility and Generalizability of the Yale Pharyngeal Residue Severity Rating Scale

Since the anatomical definitions used by the Yale Pharyngeal Residue Severity Scale are discrete, i.e., not continuous and image based, the severity rating is not affected by age, gender, or body habitus. For example, mild vallecula residue is defined as "epiglottic ligament visible." The shape and size of the vallecula are unimportant. As long as the epiglottic ligament is visible, the severity rating is mild residue. This generalizability makes it possible to determine pharyngeal residue severity for any given individual and allows the clinician to use the scale with absolute confidence. In other words, since the patient serves as their own control, there is no need to compare residue severity to another individual. Rather, the clinician compares their patient's residue severity against the reliable and validated images from the Yale Pharyngeal Residue Severity Scale.

Research and Clinical Uses

The Yale Pharyngeal Residue Severity Rating Scale can be used for both clinical advantages and research opportunities. Clinically, clinicians can now accurately classify vallecula and pyriform sinus residue severity as none, trace, mild, moderate, or severe for diagnostic purposes, determination of functional therapeutic change, and precise dissemination of shared information. Future research uses include tracking outcome measures for clinical trials investigating various swallowing interventions, demonstrating efficacy of specific interventions to reduce pharyngeal residue, determining morbidity and mortality associated with pharyngeal residue severity in different patient populations, and improving the training and accuracy of FEES interpretation by students and clinicians. We eagerly anticipate the work from clinicians around the world as they report on their use of the Yale Pharyngeal

Residue Severity Rating Scale with the dual goals of promoting patient care and documenting research success.

Summary

This book covers all aspects of pharyngeal residue severity rating. This includes comprehensive foundational information on embryology and anatomy of the pharynx, a systematic review detailing the strengths and weaknesses of all published pharyngeal residue severity rating scales to date, the original publication of the Yale Pharyngeal Residue Severity Rating Scale, a historical discussion concerning over 100 years of thoughts on the role of the epiglottis in swallowing, and a small investigation that showed exactly how easy it was for even novice, untrained, and nonmedical individuals to use the Yale Pharyngeal Residue Severity Rating Scale correctly.

References

1. Murray J, Langmore SE, Ginsberg S, Dostie A. The significance of oropharyngeal secretions and swallowing frequency in predicting aspiration. Dysphagia. 1996;11:99–103.
2. Pearson WG, Molfenter SM, Smith ZM, Steele CM. Image-based measurement of post-swallow residue: the normalized residue ratio scale. Dysphagia. 2013;28:167–77.
3. Logemann J. Evaluation and treatment of swallowing disorders. 2nd ed. Austin: Pro-Ed; 1998.
4. Perlman AL, Grayback JP, Booth BM. The relationship of vallecular residue to oral involvement, reduced hyoid elevation, and epiglottic function. J Speech Hear Res. 1992;35:734–41.
5. Dejaeger E, Pelemans W, Ponette E, Joosten E. Mechanisms involved in postdeglutition retention in the elderly. Dysphagia. 1997;12:63–7.
6. Kahrilas PJ. Pharyngeal structure and function. Dysphagia. 1993;8:303–7.
7. Langmore SE, Schatz K, Olsen N. Fiberoptic endoscopic examination of swallowing safety: a new procedure. Dysphagia. 1988;2:216–9.

8. Langmore SE. Scoring a FEES examination. In: Langmore SE, editor. Endoscopic evaluation and treatment of swallowing disorders. New York: Thieme; 2001.

9. Kelly AM, Leslie P, Beale T, Payten C, Drinnan MJ. Fibreoptic endoscopic evaluation of swallowing and videofluoroscopy: does examination type influence perception of pharyngeal severity? Clin Otolaryngol. 2006;31:425–32.

10. Leder SB, Judson BL, Sliwinski E, Madson L. Promoting safe swallowing when puree Is swallowed without aspiration but thin liquid is aspirated: nectar is enough. Dysphagia. 2013;28:58–62.

11. Neubauer PD, Rademaker AW, Leder SB. The Yale pharyngeal residue severity rating scale: an anatomically defined and image-based tool. Dysphagia. 2015;30:521–8.

12. Farneti D. Pooling score: an endoscopic model for evaluating severity of dysphagia. Acta Otorhinological Ital. 2008;28: 135–40.

13. Tohara H, Nakane A, Murata S, Mikushi S, Ouchi Y, Wakasugi Y, Takashima M, Chiba Y, Uematsu H. Inter- and inter-rater reliability in fiberoptic endoscopic evaluation of swallowing. J Oral Rehabil. 2010;37:884–91.

14. Kaneoka AS, Langmore SE, Krisciunas GP, Field K, Scheel R, McNally E, Walsh MJ, O'Dea MB, Cabral H. The Boston Residue and Clearance Scale: preliminary reliability and validity testing. Folia Phoniatr Logop. 2014;65:312–7.

15. Donzelli J, Brady S, Wesling M, Craney M. Predictive value of accumulated oropharyngeal secretions for aspiration during video nasal endoscopic evaluation of the swallow. Ann Otol Rhinol. 2003;112:469–75.

16. Han TR, Paik NJ, Park JW. Quantifying swallowing function after stroke: a functional dysphagia scale based on videofluoroscopic studies. Arch Phys Med Rehabil. 2001;82:677–82.

17. Eisenhuber E, Schima W, Schober E, Pokieser P, Stadler A, Scharitzer M, Oschatz E. Videofluoroscopic assessment of patients with dysphagia: pharyngeal retention is a predictive factor for aspiration. AJR Am J Roentgenol. 2002;178:393–8.

18. Logemann JA, Williams RB, Rademaker A, Pauloski BR, Lazarus CL, Cook I. The relationship between observations and measures of oral and pharyngeal residue from videofluorography and scintigraphy. Dysphagia. 2005;20:226–31.

19. Dyer JC, Leslie P, Drinnan MJ. Objective computer-based assessment of valleculae residue: is it useful? Dysphagia. 2008;23:7–15.

Chapter 2
Embryology and Anatomy of the Oral Cavity and Pharynx

Introduction

Knowledge of the development of the human pharynx, the complicated structure it becomes, and its crucial role in deglutition is necessary to understand the foundational underpinnings of a functional swallow. This chapter details the embryology of the branchial apparatus. The anatomy is reviewed in the order in which a food bolus would make contact, starting at the oral cavity and ending at the hypopharynx, just before the food bolus enters the esophagus. In addition, the two major postnatal developments that occur in the upper aerodigestive tract are described. Finally, prior to the more comprehensive discussion found in Chap. 5, basic information on the normal epiglottis, the pseudoepiglottis that develops after total laryngectomy, and the volume of liquid the adult hypopharynx can hold are discussed.

Embryology of the Oral Cavity and Pharynx

The oral cavity and pharynx arise embryologically from the branchial apparatus, which appears in the 4th–5th week of human development. The branchial apparatus consists of four ectodermal branchial clefts located externally in the embryologic foregut, which is the most cranial part of the

S.B. Leder, P.D. Neubauer, *The Yale Pharyngeal Residue Severity Rating Scale*, DOI 10.1007/978-3-319-29899-3_2,
© Springer International Publishing Switzerland 2016

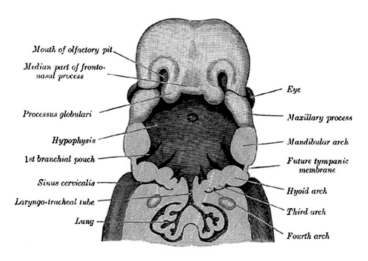

Figure 2.1 The head and neck of the human embryo, including the branchial apparatus (From Gray [6])

embryo. The embryonic pharynx forms five pharyngeal pouches internally in the foregut. The first four pouches correspond to branchial clefts externally. Between these paired clefts and pouches are five mesodermal branchial arches [1]. The pouches penetrate the mesenchymal embryonic arches but do not communicate with the clefts, thereby distinguishing themselves from gills found in amphibians and fish [2].

After formation, the branchial clefts begin to obliterate after the fifth week of development. The exception is the first cleft which becomes the external auditory canal (Fig. 2.1). The corresponding pharyngeal pouch becomes the tubotympanic recess or Eustachian tube and middle ear. The area between the pouch and the cleft becomes the tympanic membrane. The remaining four clefts obliterate by the seventh week. Those that persist become branchial cleft cysts, sinuses, or fistulae [1].

The pharyngeal pouches are associated with adult head and neck structures. The epithelial lining of the second pouch forms buds which penetrate the surrounding mesenchyme.

These buds are invaded by mesenchymal tissue to form the palatine tonsils. The second pouch persists as the palatine tonsillar fossa. The third pouch is near the superior pyriform sinus and becomes the inferior parathyroid glands and thymus [2]. The fourth pouch is at the apex or inferior extent of the pyriform sinus and becomes the superior parathyroid glands and the ultimobranchial body. The later are, in turn, incorporated by the thyroid gland to become calcitonin-secreting parafollicular C cells [2]. The fifth and sixth pouches may correspond with the laryngeal ventricle [1].

The five mesenchymal branchial arches consist of mesenchymal tissue covered by surface ectoderm and are lined internally by endoderm. Neural crest cells contribute to each arch and become part of the skeletal components of the face. The mesoderm gives rise to each arch's musculature and each arch has its own cranial nerve. Also, each arch has its own arterial component [2, 3].

The first branchial arch consists of a dorsal portion, termed the maxillary process, and a ventral portion, termed the mandibular process [4]. The maxillary process becomes the premaxilla, maxilla, and zygomatic bone. The mandibular process contains Meckel's cartilage and becomes the incus and the malleus. The mandible forms from the tissue surrounding Meckel's cartilage. The trigeminal nerve innervates the musculature of the first branchial arch. This includes the muscles of mastication, i.e., the medial and lateral pterygoids, temporalis, and masseter muscles, as well as the anterior belly of the digastric, mylohyoid, tensor tympani, and tensor veli palatini muscles [2, 3]. Derivatives of the first arch also form part of the anterior two-thirds of the tongue [4]. (See Table 2.1 for easy summary viewing of branchial arches and associated bones, cartilages, nerves, and muscles.)

The second arch includes Reichert's cartilage and gives rise to the stapes, styloid process, stylohyoid ligament, and the lesser horn and upper part of the body of the hyoid bone. The facial nerve innervates the muscles of the second arch. These muscles include the muscles of the facial expression, stapedius, stylohyoid, posterior belly of digastric, and auricular muscles [2, 3].

TABLE 2.1 Branchial arch derivatives

Branchial arch	Bone and cartilage	Nerve	Muscles
1	Premaxilla, maxilla, zygomatic bone, Meckel's cartilage (malleus and incus), mandible	Trigeminal	Tensor veli palatini, tensor tympani, masseter, medial and lateral pterygoids, temporalis, mylohyoid, posterior belly of digastric
2	Stapes, styloid process, lesser horn and upper part of hyoid bone, stylohyoid ligament	Facial	Facial expression, posterior belly of digastric, stapedius, stylohyoid
3	Greater horn and upper part of the body of the hyoid	Glossopharyngeal	Stylopharyngeus
4–6	Thyroid, cricoid, arytenoid, corniculate, and cuneiform cartilages	Fourth: Vagus (superior laryngeal)	Fourth: cricothyroid, levator palatini, pharyngeal constrictors
		Sixth: Vagus (recurrent laryngeal)	Sixth: intrinsic laryngeal

The cartilage of the third branchial arch becomes the greater horn and lower portion of the body of the hyoid bone. The glossopharyngeal nerve innervates the muscles of the third branchial arch, i.e., the stylopharyngeus muscles [2, 3]. Additionally, mesoderm from the third and fourth arches forms the posterior one-third of the tongue [4].

The cartilage of the fourth and sixth arches fuses to become the thyroid, cricoid, arytenoid, corniculate, and cuneiform cartilages of the larynx. The muscles of the fourth arch are supplied by the superior laryngeal branch of the vagus nerve and include the cricothyroid muscle, levator palatini muscle, and constrictor muscles of the pharynx. The muscles of the sixth arch are innervated by the recurrent laryngeal nerve and include the intrinsic muscles of the larynx [2, 3].

Anatomy of the Upper Aerodigestive Tract

Anatomy

The upper aerodigestive tract begins at the lips and the nasal vestibule and extends inferiorly to the subglottis and the level of the cricoid cartilage where the esophagus begins. Sagittal views of the upper aerodigestive tract are shown in both the traditional two-dimensional (Fig. 2.2) and computer-generated 3-D images (Fig. 2.3). The upper aerodigestive tract serves an overlay function as it is integral to breathing, swallowing, and speaking [4, 5]. The upper aerodigestive tract's subsites, through which the food bolus travels, are the oral cavity, oropharynx, and hypopharynx. The larynx also has a triple overlay function of preventing the food bolus from entering the airway, respiration, and verbal communication.

The Oral Cavity

The oral cavity begins at the vermillion border of the lips and extends posteriorly to the junction of the hard and soft palates superiorly and the circumvallate papillae inferiorly. The

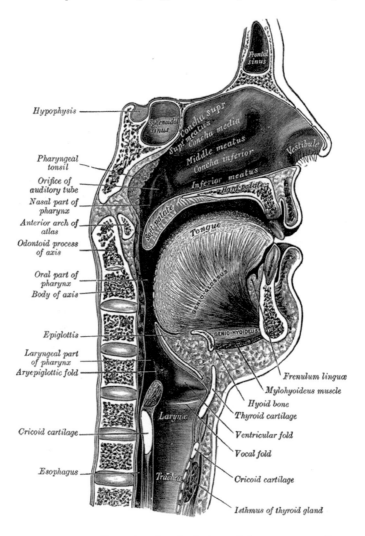

FIGURE 2.2 Two-dimensional sagittal view of the upper aerodigestive tract (From Gray [6])

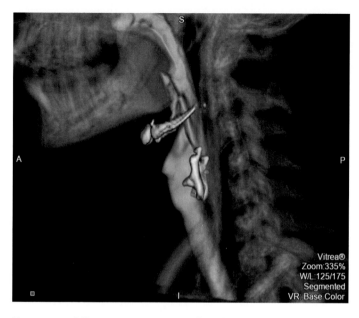

FIGURE 2.3 3-D computer-generated sagittal view of the upper aerodigestive tract

subsites of the oral cavity are the lips, oral tongue, floor of the mouth, hard palate, buccal mucosa, upper and lower alveolar ridges, and the retromolar trigone (Fig. 2.4). The retromolar trigone is a triangular area of mucosa covering the ascending ramus of the mandible [5].

The oral cavity includes ducts of the major salivary glands. Stensen's duct drains the parotid glands and enters on the buccal mucosa across from the second superior molar. Wharton's duct drains the submandibular glands and enters on the floor of the mouth lateral to the lingual frenulum [6].

The permanent teeth consist of the incisors, which are for cutting; canines, which are for tearing food; and the premolars and molars, which are used for chewing. The adult has 32 permanent teeth [4, 7].

The anterior and middle portions of the mobile oral tongue, in addition to taste sensation and speech articulation

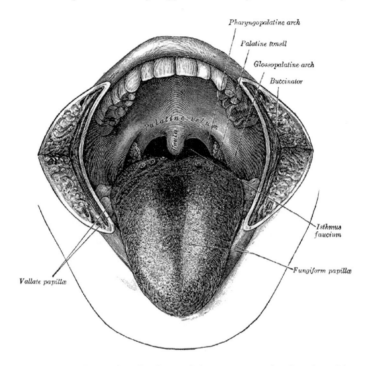

FIGURE 2.4 The oral cavity, base of the tongue, and soft palate. The cheeks have been incised and the tongue pulled forward (From Gray [6])

abilities, are critical for anterior-to-posterior oral bolus transport. The tongue consists mostly of muscle fibers. The extrinsic muscles of the tongue connect to the mandible (via the genioglossus muscle), hyoid bone (via the hyoglossus muscle), styloid processes (via the styloglossus muscle), and soft palate (via the palatoglossus muscle) and also form part of the floor of the mouth. All of the extrinsic tongue muscles are innervated by the hypoglossal nerve, except the palatoglossus which is innervated by the vagus nerve. On the back and in the midline of the dorsal surface of the tongue is the foramen cecum. Anterior and lateral from the depression of the foramen cecum are the circumvallate papillae, which separate the

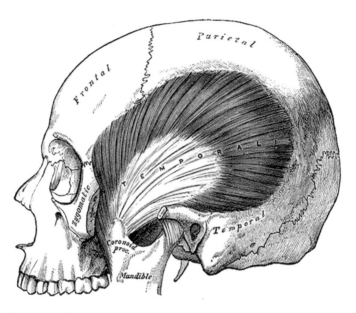

FIGURE 2.5 Temporalis muscle (From Gray [6])

oral cavity from the oropharynx. The foramen cecum is the superior end of the thyroglossal duct, from which the thyroid gland develops [6–8].

The muscles of mastication are responsible for rotary motion of the mandible in order to chew the food bolus. These muscles are the temporalis, masseter, and medial pterygoid and lateral pterygoid. The temporalis arises from the temporal fossa and inserts into the coronoid process of the mandible and is responsible for elevating and retracting the jaw (Fig. 2.5). The masseter originates from the zygoma and zygomatic process of the maxilla and inserts on the lateral mandible at the angle, and it contracts to elevate the mandible. The medial pterygoid inserts on the medial surface of the angle of the mandible and originates from the medial side of the lateral pterygoid plate and also elevates the jaw. Lastly, the lateral pterygoid originates in the lateral side of

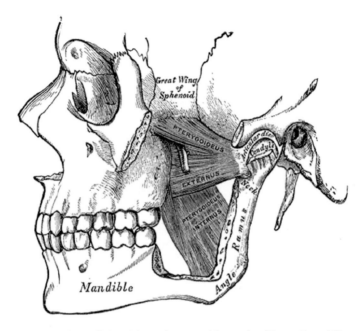

FIGURE 2.6 Medial and lateral pterygoid muscles (From Gray [6])

the lateral pterygoid plate and inserts below the condyle of the mandible and is responsible for depressing and protracting the mandible to open the mouth (Fig. 2.6). The muscles of mastication are innervated by the mandibular branch of the trigeminal nerve [4, 6–8]

The Oropharynx

As the food bolus exits the oral cavity, it enters the oropharynx, which begins at the circumvallate papillae inferiorly and the junction of the hard palate and soft palate superiorly and extends inferiorly to the hyoid bone. The subsites of the oropharynx are the palatine tonsils, base of the tongue, soft palate, and lateral and posterior pharyngeal walls [5].

The glossotonsillar sulcus is an area between the tonsil and the base of the tongue which allows for the normal flow of saliva from the oral cavity to the oropharynx [9]. The pillars of the fauces start at the anterior and posterior aspects of the soft palate and extend inferiorly on either side of the palatine tonsil. The palatoglossal muscle makes up the anterior arch and the palatopharyngeal arch comprises the posterior arch. Some fibers of the palatopharyngeus run posteriorly and form a sphincter along with the superior constrictor to form Passavant's ridge, which makes contact with the soft palate during swallowing, thereby preventing reflux of the bolus into the nasopharynx [6, 7].

The soft palate contains the tensor veli palatini muscle, levator palatini, and the musculus uvulae (Fig. 2.7). The tensor veli palatini muscle originates at the base of the medial pterygoid and inserts into the palatine aponeurosis after hooking around the pterygoid hamulus. It tenses the soft palate before elevation. The levator palatini arises from the petrous temporal bone and the medial aspect of the Eustachian tube and inserts in the palatine aponeurosis. Upon swallowing, the levator veli palatini facilitates the opening of the Eustachian tube. The musculus uvulae tenses and shortens the uvula which hangs from the midline of the soft palate in a dependent manner [6, 7].

The three constrictor muscles contain the pharynx (Fig. 2.8). The superior constrictor muscle originates at the medial pterygoid plate and mandible, the middle constrictor originates at the hyoid bone, and the inferior constrictor attaches to the thyroid and cricoid cartilages. All three constrictors insert posteriorly in a fibrous median raphe [6–8]. The constrictor muscles overlap with each other with the middle constrictor overlying the superior constrictor and underlying the inferior constrictor [6]. Between the superior and middle constrictors passes the stylopharyngeus, which originates at the styloid process and inserts in the pharyngeal musculature and the thyroid cartilage. Beginning at the base of the skull and extending inferior between the mucous membrane and muscular wall of the pharynx is the pharyngobasilar fascia.

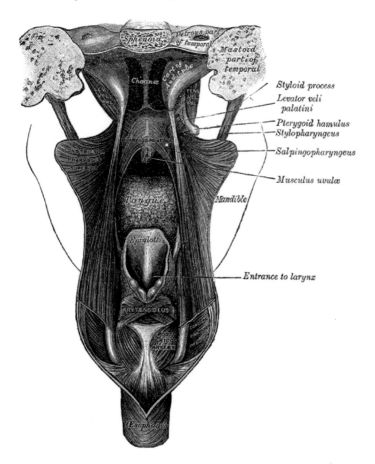

FIGURE 2.7 Posterior view of the upper aerodigestive tract (From Gray [6])

As the food bolus enters the pharynx, the stylopharyngeus elevates and widens the pharynx due to the relative lateral location of the styloid process compared the insertion at the pharyngeal musculature and thyroid cartilage. Simultaneously, the base of the tongue and larynx are drawn anteriorly and superiorly which increases the anteroposterior diameter. Once the bolus is in the pharynx, the constrictor muscles

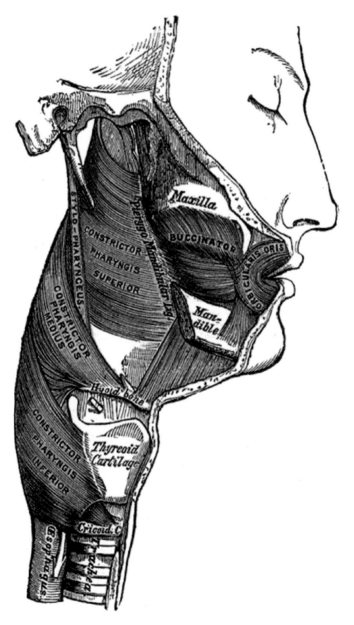

FIGURE 2.8 The constrictor muscles (From Gray [6])

contract to aid propulsion of the bolus toward the upper esophageal sphincter and esophagus [6].

The innervation of the pharynx is mainly from the pharyngeal plexus which lies on the posterior surface of the middle constrictor muscle. It contains a sensory branch from the glossopharyngeal nerve, a motor branch from the vagus nerve, and a branch of the sympathetic trunk. All of the muscles of the palate and the pharynx are supplied by this plexus, except the stylopharyngeus muscle, which is supplied by the glossopharyngeal nerve and the tensor veli palatini, which is supplied by the mandibular division of the trigeminal nerve [6, 7].

As the food bolus continues its downward path toward the esophagus, it encounters the epiglottis, which projects upward behind the base of the tongue and passively retroverts and closes over the larynx during swallowing [7]. The vallecula is the space between the base of the tongue and the epiglottis where residue may collect [10]. (See Chap. 4 for additional information on the vallecula.) Posteriorly and inferiorly from the epiglottis are the aryepiglottic folds which extend to the arytenoid cartilages. On the posterior surface of the epiglottis is the tubercle of the epiglottis which extends posterior in the midline [7].

The Epiglottis

The epiglottis is the most prominent structure in the pharynx, and no discussion of the pharynx can be complete without a description of the anatomy and physiology of the epiglottis. Anatomically, the epiglottis is a stalklike structure made of fibroelastic cartilage which overhangs the entrance to the larynx. It takes its origin from the angle of the thyroid cartilage just inferior to the thyroid notch. The thyroepiglottic, or more commonly the epiglottic ligament, serves as its attachment to the thyroid cartilage. The epiglottis presents with an anterior or lingual surface and posterior or laryngeal surface. The epiglottis can present in many different sizes, ranging from small and narrow to large and wide, and shapes, described as fanlike, leaflike, and omega. Whether it "guards" the entrance or serves as a conduit for directing bolus flow laterally to the pyriform sinuses or both has long been an area of controversy. One thing for sure, however, is that it allows the formation of a vallecula space at the base of the tongue, the lingual surface of which allows for the collection of small amounts of liquid and masticated food after the initial swallow [11]. Chapter 4 and 5 contain additional detailed information on the important role the vallecula plays in swallowing. (Parenthetically, without this vallecula space, this book would not have been possible!)

The epiglottis has no internal musculature. Physiologically, its movement is dependent on and interactive with the movement of surrounding structures. Epiglottic downfolding and rebounding to its natural resting position have been elucidated via computer modeling. Specifically, computer-based radiographic imaging analysis revealed that epiglottic downfolding during swallowing in adult man is comprised of two distinct processes [12]. The first epiglottic movement occurs at the attachment of the epiglottis to the thyroid cartilage and brings the epiglottis from its semi-vertical resting position to a horizontal orientation concurrently with elevation of the larynx and hyoid bone during swallowing. The second epiglottic movement occurs as the bolus passes through the larynx and brings the upper one-third of the epiglottis below the horizontal plane. Post-deglutitive descent of the larynx and hyoid bone allows the epiglottis to return passively to its pre-swallow, natural, and upright position.

Pseudoepiglottis Development After Total Laryngectomy

A pouch-like recess sometimes develops post-total laryngectomy and can be either a thin band or a more broadly based mass [13]. The pouch appears to result from separation of the edges of the pharyngeal closure precisely where it joins the base of the tongue. This opening allows liquid and food to enter the space under the skin flap and results in either a permanent pouch, termed a "pseudoepiglottis" or a salivary fistula [13]. When the posterior wall of the pouch is prominent, it appears similar to an epiglottis, hence the term pseudoepiglottis [13]. Radiological examination confirmed pouch location as on the anterior wall of the pharynx at its junction with the base of the tongue [14]. The average size of the pouch was reported to be 10.2 mm [15] and with a capacity of between 1 cc and 30 cc volume of liquid [13]. Fortunately, since prandial aspiration cannot occur post-total laryngectomy, the only potential risk is post-swallow dysfunction due to regurgitation of retained material.

The Hypopharynx

As the food bolus traverses to the level of the hyoid bone, it enters the hypopharynx, which is continuous and seamless with the oropharynx. The hypopharynx extends inferiorly behind the larynx to the cricopharyngeus muscle. The subsites of the hypopharynx include the posterior pharyngeal wall, pyriform sinuses, and post-cricoid area. In the hypopharynx, below the arytenoids is the anterior wall of the pharynx which is the posterior border of the larynx. This wall consists of the cricoid cartilage, the arytenoid cartilages, and the lamina of the thyroid cartilage. Between the lamina of the thyroid cartilage and the aryepiglottic folds are the pyriform sinuses, another key area (in addition to the vallecula) where residue may collect [7, 10]. (See Chap. 4 for additional discussion of the role the pyriform sinuses play in swallowing.) (And, as with the vallecula, without the pyriform sinuses, this book would not have been possible!)

The food bolus continues to be propelled downward, by the base-of-tongue driving force, to the upper esophageal sphincter which is made primarily from the cricopharyngeus muscle but also includes the inferior constrictor. It is tonically active but relaxes to allow the food bolus transit into the proximal esophagus. The vagus nerve supplies the major innervation to the upper esophageal sphincter [4, 6, 7].

How Much Volume of Liquid Can the Hypopharynx Hold?

Laryngeal penetration and tracheal aspiration of pre-swallow spillage and post-swallow food residue in the pharynx are dependent upon the volume of material that the pharynx can safely accommodate prior to overflowing into the airway. Two studies from the 1990s investigated the amount of residue remaining in the pharynx after a swallow. Cook et al. [16] used scintigraphy to measure the amount of residue after drinking a 5 mL and 10 mL bolus in two groups of normal participants. Group 1 was younger (mean age, 28 years), and group 2 was older (mean age, 68 years). Group 1 exhibited approximately 2 % bolus residue in the pharynx, while group 2 left up to approximately 13 % of the bolus in the pharynx. Dejaeger et al. [17] used VFSS to subjectively rate pharyngeal residue in normal elderly participants (mean age, 80 years) after drinking three 10 mL boluses and found 24/75 (32 %) exhibited diffuse pharyngeal residue, 15/75 (20 %) exhibited vallecula residue, 13/75 (17 %) exhibited pyriform sinus residue, while the remaining 23/75 (31 %) exhibited no visible residue.

In a series of elegant experiments, Dua et al. [18, 19] investigated the airway protective function of aerodigestive reflexes by perfusing water into the hypopharynx at the rate of 1 mL/min. Subjects were 15 healthy, adult, nonsmokers (7 M/8 F; mean age, 24.2 years ± 3.3 years). At a certain volume, the fluid level in the valleculae and pyriform sinuses triggered an irrepressible swallow called the reflexive pharyngeal swallow. The interaction of fluid volume triggering a pharyngeal swallow was termed the hypopharyngeal safe volume and operationally defined as the maximum volume of water that can safely dwell in the hypopharynx before spilling into the larynx. The threshold volume to trigger a reflexive pharyngeal swallow in all 15 subjects without topical anesthesia was 0.71 ± 0.07 mL of water. After topical pharyngeal anesthesia, in these same subjects, the volume averaged 0.61 ± 0.06 mL of water.

The reader should keep these small volumes in mind when the graded severity ratings of the Yale Pharyngeal Residue

Severity Rating Scale are discussed in Chap. 4. The volume capacity of both the valleculae and pyriform sinuses is small. This is very important because even the most experienced endoscopist must remember that the anatomically defined and image-based severity ratings are dependent upon small volumes of residue. And these small volumes potentially have large consequences for either a functionally successful or unsuccessful pharyngeal swallow.

Postnatal Development of the Oral Cavity and Pharynx

Two major changes occur in the oral cavity and pharynx during development: the descent of the epiglottis and larynx and the eruption of teeth [4]. In infancy, the epiglottis is located high in the upper airway, thereby allowing fluids to pass safely on either side of the nasopharynx and larynx, i.e., without making contact with the airway, and reducing the risk of aspiration as the bolus flows into the esophagus. This anatomical configuration makes infants obligate nasal breathers. The position of the epiglottis in other mammals is similar to that of infants. Animal studies support that the epiglottis also allows inspired air through the nose to be closed off from the oral cavity, perhaps enhancing olfaction. The epiglottis and larynx descend in the pharynx between 4 and 6 months of age [20]. This descent enables airflow through the oral cavity and pharynx, ultimately allowing for voice and speech production, but increasing the risk of prandial aspiration [4]. (See Chap. 5 for additional information on the history, role, and controversy of the epiglottis in swallowing.)

The second major development change in the upper aerodigestive tract is the eruption of teeth, which begins around 7 months of age. By two-and-a-half years of age, there are 20 deciduous teeth, consisting of 8 incisors, 4 canines, and 8 molars. By the age of six, these teeth begin to fall out and are replaced with permanent dentition, starting with the eruption of the lower first permanent molars. This mixed dentition phase is variable and can last up to the teenage years [21].

Conclusion

A firm grasp of the intricate embryology, anatomy, and maturational development of the oral and pharyngeal structures involved with swallowing in the upper aerodigestive tract is foundational to the diagnosis and treatment of swallowing disorders. Starting with the branchial apparatus at 5 weeks of gestation and continuing to the developmental changes in early adulthood, the complicated structure of the oral cavity and pharynx begets its life-sustaining function.

References

1. Skandalakis JE, Gray SW. Embryology for surgeons: the embryological basis for the treatment of congenital defects. Philadelphia: Saunders; 1972.
2. Sadler TW, Langman J. Langman's medical embryology. Philadelphia: Lippincott Williams & Wilkins; 2004.
3. Moore KL, Persaud TVN, Torchia MG. The developing human: clinically oriented embryology. Philadelphia: Saunders/Elsevier; 2008.
4. German R, Palmer J. Anatomy and development of the oral cavity and pharynx. GI Motility Online. 2006.
5. Deschler DG, Moore MG, Smith RV, editors. Quick reference guide to TNM staging of head and neck cancer and neck dissection classification. 4th ed. Alexandria: American Academy of Otolaryngology–Head and Neck Surgery Foundation; 2014.
6. Gray H. Anatomy of the human body. Philadelphia: Lea & Febiger; 1918. www.bartleby.com/107/.
7. Aitken JT, Causey G, Joseph J, Young JZ. A manual of human anatomy, head and neck. London: E & S Livingstone LTD.; 1964.
8. "Master Muscle List." Lumen Learn 'Em. Ed. Michael Dauzvardis. Loyola University Medical Education Network, Jan.-Feb. 1996. Web. 17 Dec. 2015. www.meddean.luc.edu/lumen/meded/grossanatomy/dissector/mml/mmlalpha.htm.
9. Shin J, Cunningham MJ. Otolaryngology prep and practice. Plural Publishing; San Diego, CA. 2012.
10. Murray J, Langmore SE, Ginsberg S, et al. The significance of oropharyngeal secretions and swallowing frequency in predicting aspiration. Dysphagia. 1996;11:99–103.

11. Kirchner JA. Physiology of the larynx. 3rd ed. Washington: American Academy of Otolaryngology–Head and Neck Surgery Foundation, Inc; 1986.
12. Vandaele DJ, Perlman AL, Cassell MD. Intrinsic fibre architecture and attachments of the human epiglottis and their contributions to the mechanism of deglutition. J Anat. 1995;186:1–15.
13. Kirchner JA, Scatliff JH, Dey FL, Shedd DP. The pharynx after laryngectomy. Laryngoscope. 1963;73:18–33.
14. Davis RK, Vincent ME, Shapshay SM, Strong MS. The anatomy and complications of "T" versus vertical closure of the hypopharynx after laryngectomy. Laryngosocpe. 1982;92:16–20.
15. Nayar RC, Sharma VP, Arora MML. A study of the pharynx after laryngectomy. J Laryngol Otol. 1984;98:807–10.
16. Cook IJ, Weltman MD, Wallace K, Shaw DW, McKay E, Butler SP. Influence of aging on oral-pharyngeal bolus transit and clearance during swallowing: scintigraphic study. Am J Physiol. 1994; 266:G972–7.
17. Dejaeger E, Pelemans W, Ponette E, Joosten E. Mechanisms involved in postdeglutition retention in the elderly. Dysphagia. 1997;12:63–7.
18. Dua K, Surapaneni SN, Kuribayashi S, Hafeezullah SR. Protective role of aerodigestive reflexes against aspiration: study on subjects with impaired and preserved reflexes. Gastroenterology. 2011;140:1927–33.
19. Dua K, Surapaneni SN, Kuribayashi S, Hafeezullah SR. Pharyngeal airway protective reflexes are triggered before the maximum volume of fluid that the hypopharynx can safely hold is exceeded. Am J Physiol Gastrointest Liver Physiol. 2011;301:G197–202.
20. Sasaki CT, Levine PA, Laitman JT, Crelin Jr ES. Postnatal descent of the epiglottis in man. A preliminary report. Arch Otolaryngol. 1977;103(3):169–71.
21. Thomson K, Dean T, Marks M. Paediatric handbook. 8th ed. Blackwell Publishing; Hoboken, NJ. 2009.

Chapter 3
A Systematic Literature Review of Pharyngeal Residue Severity Rating Scales Based on Fiberoptic Endoscopic Evaluation of Swallowing

Introduction

Identification of pharyngeal residue and its severity have been primary goals of the fiberoptic endoscopic evaluation of swallowing (FEES) since the procedure's initial description [1]. Sensitivity and specificity for determination of presence or absence of pharyngeal residue during FEES were good [2], and the importance of this key component has been corroborated by subsequent state-of-the-art reports [3–5]. Over the past three decades, FEES has become a widely used objective instrumental examination to diagnose pharyngeal phase dysphagia, implement therapeutic interventions, and make recommendations for safe oral alimentation [6–10]. However, a reliable, validated, and generalizable pharyngeal residue severity rating scale for FEES has been lacking.

Neubauer PD, Hersey DP, Leder SB. Pharyngeal residue severity rating scales based on fiberoptic endoscopic evaluation of swallowing: A systematic review. Dysphagia. 2016;30:521–8. doi:10.1007/s00455-015-9682-6 (Used and modified with kind permission from Springer Science + Business Media).

S.B. Leder, P.D. Neubauer, *The Yale Pharyngeal Residue Severity Rating Scale*, DOI 10.1007/978-3-319-29899-3_3,
© Springer International Publishing Switzerland 2016

Pharyngeal residue is a clinical sign of potential prandial aspiration [11]. An accurate description of pharyngeal residue severity is, therefore, an important but difficult clinical challenge [12]. Many studies have reported findings of pharyngeal residue during FEES, but no attempt was made to determine pharyngeal residue severity patterns [6, 8, 13–43]. Simply stating that vallecula and pyriform sinus residue occurred is not helpful for either clinical or research purposes as patient information cannot be shared and efficacy of treatment interventions cannot be determined. The absence of a reliable, validated, and generalizable scale to determine vallecula and pyriform sinus residue severity patterns has made it difficult for clinicians to share patient information and determine benefits of therapeutic interventions.

The purpose of this systematic review is to evaluate the published literature since 1995 that investigated pharyngeal residue severity rating scales based on FEES. The research question this study addresses is: Do the qualitative and psychometric properties of published scales meet the criteria necessary for reliable, valid, and generalizable determination of vallecula and pyriform sinus pharyngeal residue severity?

Methods

Search Methodology

The following databases were searched for relevant studies: MEDLINE (OvidSP 1946–April Week 3 2015), Embase (OvidSP 1974–2015 April 20), Scopus (Elsevier), and the unindexed material in PubMed (NLM/NIH). All searches were conducted on April 20, 2015, except for Scopus, which was conducted on April 23, 2015. Supplementary efforts to identify studies included checking the reference lists of the articles retrieved.

The databases were searched using both controlled vocabulary words and synonymous free text words for the topic of interest (deglutition disorders, pharyngeal residue, endoscopy, videofluoroscopy, fiberoptic technology, food, aspirate, etc.) and the outcomes of interest (scores, scales, grades, FEES, tests, etc.). The search strategies were adjusted for the syntax appropriate for each database/platform. The search was limited to articles published since 1995 and written in the English language. See appendix for MEDLINE search strategy.

Inclusion Criteria

This systematic review focused solely on studies that reported on completed and generalizable pharyngeal residue severity rating scales based on FEES. Scales limited to a specific disease process or diagnosis were not included.

Study Selection

Titles and abstracts of the retrieved articles were independently evaluated by two reviewers (PDN and SBL). Abstracts that did not provide adequate information regarding inclusion criteria were retrieved for full-text evaluation. The reviewers independently evaluated full-text articles and determined study eligibility. Disagreements were resolved by consensus agreement.

Data Extraction

The same two reviewers independently conducted study selection and data extraction. General qualitative characteristics of the studies collected included prospective or retrospective design, year of publication, severity definitions, scale type (binary, ordinal, or estimation), number of raters, experience of raters, and number of images rated. Psychometric properties collected were test/retest times, randomization of images, intra- and inter-rater reliability, and validity statistics.

Data Analysis

A qualitative summary composed of descriptive characteristics and psychometric properties of the scales used to
evaluate pharyngeal residue severity ratings based on FEES
was created for each included study (Table 3.1). Categories
included were study design, sample size, severity definitions,
scale type, number and experience of raters, randomization
of images, and intra- and inter-rater reliability and construct
validity.

Operational Definitions

1. Pharyngeal residue was operationally defined as pre-
   swallow secretions and post-swallow food residue in the
   vallecula and pyriform sinuses not entirely cleared by a
   swallow [48].
2. The operational definition of a pharyngeal residue severity
   rating scale was reliable and valid ratings of pharyngeal
   residue severity patterns, not to determine why residue
   occurs or ascertain the timing of residue occurrence during
   swallowing.
3. Scale types were operationally defined as binary (pres-
   ence/absence of residue), ordinal (to capture progressively
   increasing amounts of residue), and estimation (amount of
   observed residue as an estimate of the percentage of the
   original bolus).
4. The valleculae were anatomically defined as the spaces
   between the base of the tongue and epiglottis [49].
5. The pyriform sinuses were anatomically defined as the
   spaces formed on both sides of the pharynx between the
   fibers of the inferior pharyngeal constrictor muscle and the
   sides of the thyroid cartilage and lined by orthogonally
   directed fibers of the palatopharyngeus muscle and pharyngobasilar fascia [49].

TABLE 3.1 Qualitative summary of the seven pharyngeal residue severity rating scales developed for general use based on FEES

Study	Study design	Total N	Severity definitions	Scale type	Number of raters	How scale is learned: Naïve	Trained	Expert	Years of experience	Randomized presentations	Intra-/inter-rater reliability	Construct validity	Test/retest
Murray et al. [11]	Retrospective cohort	69 videos	Descriptive text only	Binary	2	No	No	Yes	Not reported	No	No	No	Not reported
Donzelli et al. [44]	Prospective cohort	104 videos	Descriptive text only	Estimation	2	No	No	No	Not reported	No	Inter only	No	Not reported
Kelly et al. [9]	Prospective cohort	15 still	Descriptive text only	Ordinal	15	No	No	Yes	Not reported	Yes	Yes	No	1 week
Farneti [45]	Retrospective cohort	520 videos	Descriptive text only	Ordinal	Not reported	No	No	Yes	Not reported	No	No	No	Not reported
Tohara et al. [46]	Retrospective cohort	10 videos	Descriptive text only	Ordinal	9	No	No	Yes	Mean 5.4±1.9	Yes	Yes	No	1 week
Park et al. [47]	Retrospective cohort	50 videos	Descriptive text only	Binary/ Estimation	1	No	No	Yes	7	No	No	No	Not reported
Neubauer et al. [48]	Retrospective cohort	25 still	Descriptive text and images	Ordinal	20	Yes	Yes	Yes	Mean 8.3 Range 2 – 27	Yes	Yes	Yes	2 weeks

Results

The initial search retrieved 4,388 potentially relevant citations. A total of 2,215 duplicates were excluded. The resulting 2,173 titles and abstracts were manually reviewed and an additional 2,037 excluded. Review of the references in the full texts of the remaining 136 articles revealed two new citations. This brought the total number of articles included for eligibility assessment to 138, and after full-text reviews, a total of seven studies specific to pharyngeal residue severity rating scales based on FEES were identified for inclusion in the qualitative analysis (Fig. 3.1).

Pharyngeal Residue Severity Rating Scales Based on FEES

A qualitative summary of the descriptive characteristics and psychometric properties of the seven pharyngeal residue severity rating scales based on FEES indicated major design flaws that precluded reliable, valid, and generalizable use of 6 scales [9, 11, 44–47]. These deficiencies included inadequate number of raters, no reporting of raters' years of experience or training on scale, nonrandomization of images, and missing statistical analyses of inter- and intra-rater reliability and construct validity. Only the Yale Pharyngeal Residue Severity Rating Scale [48], an anatomically defined and image-based tool, met all criteria necessary for a valid, reliable, and generalizable vallecula and pyriform sinus residue severity rating scale based on FEES (Table 3.1). Below are synopses of each of the reviewed scales.

Accumulated Oropharyngeal Secretions

Murray et al. [11] performed a retrospective binary analysis of pharyngeal residue severity based on 69 FEES videos. A gross estimation of volume of secretions in the valleculae and pyriform sinuses was made by two expert raters without specific training in use of the scale. Years of experience for the raters were not reported, videos were not randomized, and no test/retest reliability or construct validity was performed.

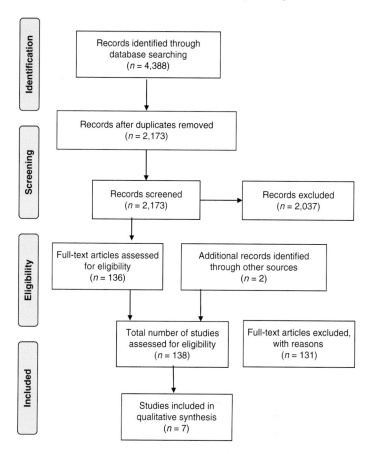

FIGURE 3.1 Flowchart of citations included in the systematic review illustrating the process through which relevant data were retrieved

Marianjoy 5-Point and 3-Point Secretion Severity Scales

Donzelli et al. [44] performed a prospective estimation analysis of pharyngeal residue severity based on 104 FEES videos and used a 5-point estimation scale of vallecula and pyriform sinus severity (normal < 10 % filled, mild 10–25 % filled, moderate > 25 % filled; severe has laryngeal penetration; profound has aspiration) and a reduced 3-point scale (functional

0–25 % filled; severe has laryngeal penetration; profound has aspiration). Two expert raters with unknown years of experience and no specific training in use of the scales participated. Videos were not randomized and only inter-rater reliability reported. A high correlation was reported for the 5-point and 3-point scales. No construct validity was reported for either the 5-point or 3-point scale.

Perception of Pharyngeal Residue Severity

Kelly et al. [9] performed a prospective ordinal analysis of pharyngeal residue severity based on 15 still FEES images and used a 5-point ordinal scale (none, coating, mild, moderate, severe). Definitions of severity were not provided. A total of 15 expert raters with unknown years of experience and no training in use of the scale participated. Videos were randomized and re-rated 1 week later by all raters. Intra-rater reliability was good, i.e., 0.72, while inter-rater reliability was moderate, i.e., 0.51. No construct validity was reported

Pooling Score

Farneti [45] performed a retrospective ordinal analysis of pharyngeal residue severity using 520 FEES videos and used a 3-point ordinal scale (coated, minimally filled, entirely filled). Definitions of severity were not provided. However, the authors did not report if all videos were analyzed. Neither the number of expert raters nor whether they were trained on use of the scale was reported. Videos were not randomized and no intra- or inter-rater reliability or construct validity was reported.

Inter- and Intra-rater Reliability with FEES

Tohara et al. [46] performed a retrospective analysis of vallecula and pyriform sinus residue severity based on 10 FEES videos chosen by a single expert with unreported years of experience and used a 3-point ordinal scale (trace, small, large). Definitions of severity were not provided. There were 9 expert raters with a mean of 5.4 (±1.9) years of experience and no training on use of the scale. Videos were randomized and re-rated four times at 1 week intervals. Overall intra-rater reliability ranged from 0.53 ± 0.04 to 0.78 ± 0.03, and inter-rater reliability ranged from 0.35 ± 0.04 to 0.46 ± 0.04. No construct validity was reported.

Detection Rates of Pharyngeal Residue

Park et al. [47] performed a retrospective binary estimation of vallecula and pyriform sinus residue severity, i.e.,>15 % filled or not, based on 50 FEES videos. There was only a single expert rater with 7 years of experience but with no training on use of the scale. No randomization of images, intra- or inter-rater reliability, or construct validity was reported.

The Yale Pharyngeal Residue Severity Rating Scale

Neubauer et al. [48] performed a retrospective, ordinal, anatomically defined, and image-based analysis of vallecula and pyriform sinus severity rating patterns based on 25 still images from FEES which corresponded to a 5-point ordinal scale (none, trace, mild, moderate, severe) (see Tables 3.2 and 3.3 for definitions of vallecula and pyriform sinus residue severity patterns, respectively). Specifically, a total of 261 FEES evaluations were reviewed, 101 images were selected, and consensus agreement between two expert judges with a combined 26 years of performing and interpreting FEES allowed for selection of 25 potential final images, i.e., a no residue exemplar and three exemplars each of trace, mild, moderate, and severe vallecula and pyriform sinus residue. Hard-copy color images of the no residue, 12 vallecula, and 12 pyriform sinus images were randomized by residue location for hierarchical categorization by 20 raters trained at 18 different institutions from around the world, i.e.,

TABLE 3.2 Definitions for severity of vallecula residue [48]

I	None	0 %	No residue
II	Trace	1–5 %	Trace coating of the mucosa
III	Mild	5–25 %	Epiglottic ligament visible
IV	Moderate	25–50 %	Epiglottic ligament covered
V	Severe	>50 %	Filled to epiglottic rim

TABLE 3.3 Definitions for severity of pyriform sinus residue [48]

I	None	0 %	No residue
II	Trace	1–5 %	Trace coating of mucosa
III	Mild	5–25 %	Up wall to quarter full
IV	Moderate	25–50 %	Up wall to half full
V	Severe	>50 %	Filled to aryepiglottic fold

otolaryngology residents ($n = 11$), attending otolaryngologists ($n = 5$), speech-language pathologists ($n = 3$), and physician assistant ($n = 1$). The raters had different durations of experience in performing and interpreting FEES evaluations (mean 8.3 years, range 2–27 years). Raters were grouped by years of FEES experience and training status. Years of experience indicated that 10 raters had ≤4 years (mean 2.8 years, range 2–4 years) and 10 raters had ≥5 years (mean 13.4 years, range 5–27 years). Training was done once, with random assignment of 10 raters to receive and 10 raters not to receive pre-rating training in determining vallecula and pyriform sinus pharyngeal residue severity ratings. Training included written definitions, visual depictions, verbal explanations, and clarifying questions/answers of the severity ratings. No training was limited to only written definitions and visual depictions of the severity ratings. Intra-rater test-retest reliability, inter-rater reliability, and construct validity for severity ratings for all images were performed by the same two expert judges and 20 raters, 2 weeks apart, and with the order of image presentations randomized. Analyses were done separately for vallecula and pyriform sinus locations. Residue ratings were excellent for intra-rater reliability for vallecula (kappa = 0.957 + 0.014) and pyriform sinus (kappa = 0.854 ± 0.021), very good to excellent for inter-rater reliability for vallecula (kappa = 0.868 ± 0.011) and pyriform sinus (kappa = 0.751 ± 0.011), and excellent for validity for vallecula (kappa = 0.951 ± 0.014) and pyriform sinus (kappa = 0.908 ± 0.017) locations. More years of experience did not result in higher kappa values for either vallecula ($p = 0.20$) or pyriform sinus ($p = 0.23$) residue ratings. Training did not result in higher kappa values for either vallecula ($p = 0.17$) or pyriform sinus ($p = 0.55$) residue ratings.

Discussion

This is the first report to systematically review the qualitative and psychometric properties of pharyngeal residue severity rating scales based on FEES. A summary of the qualitative characteristics and psychometric properties of the 7 pharyngeal residue severity rating scales based on FEES found methodological deficiencies that precluded reliable, valid, and generalizable use of 6 scales [9, 11, 44–47]. These deficiencies included lack of clear definitions, inadequate sample size and number of raters, no reporting of raters' years of experience or training on scale, nonrandomization of images, and missing statistical analyses of inter- and intra-rater reliability and construct validity.

Only the Yale Pharyngeal Residue Severity Rating Scale [48], an anatomically defined and image-based tool, met all criteria necessary for a valid, reliable, and generalizable vallecula and pyriform sinus residue severity rating scale based on FEES. For the first time, clinicians can accurately and reliably classify vallecula and pyriform sinus residue severity patterns using high-quality full-color images that correspond precisely with the severity ratings of none, trace, mild, moderate, and severe (Tables 3.2 and 3.3). Also, since no differences were found based on years of experience or prior training on use of the scale, proficiency is readily achievable in a short period of time by clinicians from different specialty areas and with different levels of expertise.

The generalizability and versatility of the Yale Pharyngeal Residue Severity Rating Scale allow for both clinical advantages and research opportunities. Clinical uses include accurate diagnosis of vallecula and pyriform sinus residue severity, assessment of functional therapeutic change, and precise dissemination of information among clinicians. Research uses include tracking the progress of outcome measures for targeted swallowing interventions, supporting efficacy of specific interventions to reduce pharyngeal residue, longitudinal determination of morbidity and mortality associated with pharyngeal residue severity patterns in different patient populations, and improving the training and accuracy of FEES interpretation by students and clinicians.

Conclusion

This systematic review investigated the qualitative and psychometric properties of pharyngeal residue severity rating scales based on FEES. There is a need for a qualitative and psychometrically reliable, validated, and generalizable pharyngeal residue severity rating scale that is anatomically specific, image-based, and easily learned by both novice and experienced clinicians. A total of seven reports were identified, but six were of poor quality and failed to employ adequate qualitative and psychometric methods necessary for a robust pharyngeal residue severity rating scale. Only the Yale Pharyngeal Residue Severity Rating Scale [48] met all criteria necessary for reliable, valid, and generalizable determination of vallecula and pyriform sinus pharyngeal residue severity ratings based on FEES.

Appendix. Ovid MEDLINE Search Strategies

1	exp Deglutition/
2	exp Deglutition Disorders/
3	pharyngeal residue.mp.
4	(swallow* and residue).mp.
5	1 or 2 or 3 or 4
6	Endoscopes/
7	endoscop*.mp.
8	(fiberoptic and endoscopic).mp.
9	videofluoroscop*.mp.
10	Fiber Optic Technology/
11	exp Fluoroscopy/
12	FEES.mp.
13	6 or 7 or 8 or 9 or 10 or 11 or 12
14	test*.mp.
15	evaluat*.mp.
16	scale*.mp.
17	grade*.mp.
18	score*.mp.
19	FEES.mp.
20	14 or 15 or 16 or 17 or 18 or 19
21	aspirat*.mp.
22	food/
23	food.mp.
24	swallow*.mp.
25	21 or 22 or 23or 24
26	5 and 13 and 20 and 25
27	limit 26 to (english language and yr = "1995 -Current")

References

1. Langmore SE, Schatz K, Olsen N. Fiberoptic endoscopic examination of swallowing safety: a new procedure. Dysphagia. 1988; 2:216–9.
2. Langmore S, Schatz K, Olson N. Endoscopic and videofluoroscopic evaluations of swallowing and aspiration. Ann Otol Rhinol Laryngol. 1991;100:678–81.
3. Hiss SG, Postma GN. Fiberoptic endoscopic evaluation of swallowing. Laryngoscope. 2003;113:1386–93.
4. Leder SB, Murray JT. Fiberoptic endoscopic evaluation of swallowing. Phys Med Rehabil Clin N Am. 2008;19:787–801.
5. Leder SB, Brady SL. Fiberoptic endoscopic evaluation of swallowing. In: Suiter DM, Gosa MM, editors. Dysphagia: diagnosis and treatment in children and adults. Thieme, NY (in press).
6. Wu CH, Hsiao TY, Chen JC, Chang YC, Lee SY. Evaluation of swallowing safety with fiberoptic endoscope: comparison with videofluoroscopic technique. Laryngoscope. 1997;107:396–401.
7. Leder SB, Sasaki CT, Burrell MI. Fiberoptic endoscopic evaluation of dysphagia to identify silent aspiration. Dysphagia. 1998; 13:19–21.
8. Leder SB, Karas DE. Fiberoptic endoscopic evaluation of swallowing in the pediatric population. Laryngoscope. 2000;110:1132–6.
9. Kelly AM, Leslie P, Beale T, Payten C, Drinnan MJ. Fibreoptic endoscopic evaluation of swallowing and videofluoroscopy: does examination type influence perception of pharyngeal residue severity? Clin Otolaryngol. 2006;31:425–32.
10. Kelly AM, Drinnan MJ, Leslie P. Assessing penetration and aspiration: how do videofluoroscopy and fiberoptic endoscopic evaluation of swallowing compare? Laryngoscope. 2007;117:1723–7.
11. Murray J, Langmore SE, Ginsberg S, Dostie A. The significance of accumulated oropharyngeal secretions and swallowing frequency in predicting aspiration. Dysphagia. 1996;11:99–103.
12. Pearson Jr WG, Molfenter SM, Smith ZM, Steele CM. Image-based measurement of post-swallow residue: the normalized residue ratio scale. Dysphagia. 2013;28:167–77.
13. Bastian RW. Videoendoscopic evaluation of patients with dysphagia: an adjunct to the modified barium swallow. Otolaryngol Head Neck Surg. 1991;104:339–50.
14. Barquist E, Brown M, Cohn S, Lundy D, Jackowski J. Postextubation fiberoptic endoscopic evaluation of swallowing after prolonged endotracheal intubation: a randomized, prospective trial. Crit Care Med. 2001;29:1710–3.

15. Blumin JH, Pcolinsky DE, Atkins JP. Laryngeal findings in advanced Parkinson's disease. Ann Otol Rhinol Laryngol. 2004;113:253–8.

16. Brady S, Donzelli J. The modified barium swallow and the functional endoscopic evaluation of swallowing. Otolaryngol Clin North Am. 2013;46:1009–22.

17. Clayton NA, Carnaby GD, Peters MJ, Ing AJ. Impaired laryngopharyngeal sensitivity in patients with COPD: the association with swallow function. Int J Speech Lang Pathol. 2014;16:615–23.

18. da Silva AP, Lubianca Neto JF, Santoro PP. Comparison between videofluoroscopy and endoscopic evaluation of swallowing for the diagnosis of dysphagia in children. Otolaryngol Head Neck Surg. 2010;143:204–9.

19. De Alencar Nunes MC, Jurkiewicz AL, Santos RS, Furkim AM, Massi G, Pinto GSA, Lange MC. Correlation between brain injury and dysphagia in adult patients with stroke. Int Arch Otorhinolaryngol. 2012;16:313–21.

20. De Sordi M, Mourão LF, Da Silva AA, Flosi LC. Interdisciplinary evaluation of dysphagia: clinical swallowing evaluation and videoendoscopy of swallowing. Braz J Otorhinolaryngol. 2009; 75:776–87.

21. Duval M, Black MA, Gesser R, Krug M, Ayotte D. Multidisciplinary evaluation and management of dysphagia: the role for otolaryngologists. J Otolaryngol Head Neck Surg. 2009;38:227–32.

22. Dworkin JP, Hill SL, Stachler RJ, Meleca RJ, Kewson D. Swallowing function outcomes following nonsurgical therapy for advanced-stage laryngeal carcinoma. Dysphagia. 2006;21:66–74.

23. Jensen K, Lambertsen K, Grau C. Late swallowing dysfunction and dysphagia after radiotherapy for pharynx cancer: frequency, intensity and correlation with dose and volume parameters. Radiother Oncol. 2007;85:74–82.

24. Kaye GM, Zorowitz RD, Baredes S. Role of flexible laryngoscopy in evaluating aspiration. Ann Otol Rhinol Laryngol. 1997;106:705–9.

25. Kondo E, Jinnouchi O, Ohnishi H, Kawata I, Nakano S, Goda M, Kitamura Y, Abe K, Hoshikawa H, Okamoto H, Takeda N. Effects of aural stimulation with capsaicin ointment on swallowing function in elderly patients with non-obstructive dysphagia. Clin Interv Aging. 2014;9:1661–7.

26. Leder SB. Serial fiberoptic endoscopic swallowing evaluations in the management of patients with dysphagia. Arch Phys Med Rehabil. 1998;79:1264–9.

27. Leder SB, Acton LM, Lisitano HL, Murray JT. Fiberoptic endo-scopic evaluation of swallowing (FEES) with and without blue-dyed food. Dysphagia. 2005;20:157–62.
28. Leder SB, Bayar S, Sasaki CT, Salem RR. Fiberoptic endoscopic evaluation of swallowing in assessing aspiration after transhiatal esophagectomy. J Am Coll Surg. 2007;205:581–5.
29. Leder SB, Novella S, Patwa H. Use of fiberoptic endoscopic evaluation of swallowing (FEES) in patients with amyotrophic lateral sclerosis. Dysphagia. 2004;19:177–81.
30. Leder SB, Ross DA. Incidence of vocal fold immobility in patients with dysphagia. Dysphagia. 2005;20:163–7.
31. Leder SB, Suiter DM, Duffey D, Judson BL. Vocal fold immobil-ity and aspiration status: a direct replication study. Dysphagia. 2012;27:265–70.
32. Link DT, Willging JP, Miller CK, Cotton RT, Rudolph CD. Pediatric laryngopharyngeal sensory testing during flexible endoscopic evaluation of swallowing: feasible and correlative. Ann Otol Rhinol Laryngol. 2000;109:899–905.
33. Momosaki R, Abo M, Kobayashi K. Swallowing analysis for semisolid food texture in poststroke dysphagic patients. J Stroke Cerebrovasc Dis. 2013;22:267–70.
34. Patterson M, Brain R, Chin R, Veivers D, Back M, Wignall A, Eade T. Functional swallowing outcomes in nasopharyngeal can-cer treated with IMRT at 6 to 42 months post-radiotherapy. Dysphagia. 2014;29:663–70.
35. Sakamoto T, Horiuchi A, Nakayama Y. Transnasal endoscopic evaluation of swallowing: a bedside technique to evaluate ability to swallow pureed diets in elderly patients with dysphagia. Can J Gastroenterol. 2013;27:459–62.
36. Seidl RO, Nusser-Muller-Busch R, Westhofen M, Ernst A. Oropharyngeal findings of endoscopic examination in swallowing disorders of neurological origin. Eur Arch Otorhinolaryngol. 2008;265:963–70.
37. Simons JA, Fietzek UM, Waldmann A, Warnecke T, Schuster T, Ceballos-Baumann AO. Development and validation of a new screening questionnaire for dysphagia in early stages of Parkinson's disease. Parkinsonism Relat Disord. 2014;20:992–8.
38. Sulica L, Hembree A, Blitzer A. Swallowing and sensation: evaluation of deglutition in the anesthetized larynx. Ann Otol Rhinol Laryngol. 2002;111:291–4.
39. Ulualp S, Brown A, Sanghavi R, Rivera-Sanchez Y. Assessment of laryngopharyngeal sensation in children with dysphagia. Laryngoscope. 2013;123:2291–5.

40. Valbuza JS, de Oliveira MM, Zancanella E, Conti CF, Prado LB, Carvalho LB, Do Prado GF. Swallowing dysfunction related to obstructive sleep apnea: a nasal fibroscopy pilot study. Sleep Breath. 2011;15:209–13.

41. Warnecke T, Oelenberg S, Teismann I, Suntrup S, Hamacher C, Young P, Ringelstein EB, Dziewas R. Dysphagia in X-linked bulbospinal muscular atrophy (Kennedy disease). Neuromuscul Disord. 2009;19:704–8.

42. Warnecke T, Teismann I, Zimmermann J, Oelenberg S, Ringelstein EB, Dziewas R. Fiberoptic endoscopic evaluation of swallowing with simultaneous tensilon application in diagnosis and therapy of myasthenia gravis. J Neurol. 2008;255:224–30.

43. Wu CH, Hsiao TY, Ko JY, Hsu MM. Dysphagia after radiotherapy: endoscopic examination of swallowing in patients with nasopharyngeal carcinoma. Ann Otol Rhinol Laryngol. 2000;109:320–5.

44. Donzelli J, Brady S, Wesling M, Craney M. Predictive value of accumulated oropharyngeal secretions for aspiration during video nasal endoscopic evaluation of the swallow. Ann Otol Rhinol Laryngol. 2003;112:469–75.

45. Farneti D. Pooling score: an endoscopic model for evaluating severity of dysphagia. Acta Otorhinolaryngol Ital. 2008;28: 135–40.

46. Tohara H, Nakane A, Murata S, Mikushi S, Ouchi Y, Wakasugi Y, Takashima M, Chiba Y, Uematsu H. Inter- and intra-rater reliability in fibroptic endoscopic evaluation of swallowing. J Oral Rehabil. 2010;37:884–91.

47. Park WY, Lee TH, Ham NS, Park JW, Lee YG, Cho SJ, Lee JS, Hong SJ, Jeon SR, Kim HG, Cho JY, Kim JO, Cho JH, Lee JS. Adding endoscopist-directed flexible endoscopic evaluation of swallowing to the videofluoroscopic swallowing study increased the detection rates of penetration, aspiration, and pharyngeal residue. Gut Liver. 2014;9:623–8.

48. Neubauer PD, Rademaker AW, Leder SB. The Yale Pharyngeal Residue Severity Rating Scale: an anatomically defined and image-based tool. Dysphagia. 2015;30(5):521–8. doi:10.1007/s00455-015-9631-4.

49. Logemann JA, Rademaker AW, Pauloski BR, Ohmae Y, Kahrilas PJ. Normal swallowing physiology as viewed by videofluoroscopy and videoendoscopy. Folia Phoniatr Logop. 1998;50:311–9.

Chapter 4
The Yale Pharyngeal Residue Severity Rating Scale: An Anatomically Defined and Image-Based Tool

Introduction

Pharyngeal residue, defined as pre-swallow secretions and post-swallow food residue in the pharynx not entirely cleared by a swallow, is a clinical predictor of prandial aspiration [1]. An accurate description of pharyngeal residue severity is an important but difficult clinical challenge [2]. Pharyngeal residue occurs in either the valleculae (spaces between the base of the tongue and epiglottis) or the pyriform sinuses (spaces formed on both sides of the pharynx between the fibers of the inferior pharyngeal constrictor muscle and the sides of the thyroid cartilage and lined by orthogonally directed fibers of the palatopharyngeus muscle and pharyngobasilar fascia) [3].

Different types of scales have attempted to classify pharyngeal residue, but none have demonstrated the combination of adequate reliability, interpretive validity, and ease of administration to be clinically useful. Scale examples are: (1)

Neubauer PD, Rademaker AW, Leder SB. The Yale pharyngeal residue severity rating scale: An anatomically defined and image-based tool. Dysphagia. 2015;30:521–8. doi:10.1007/s00455-015-9631-4 (Used and modified with kind permission from Springer Science + Business Media).

S.B. Leder, P.D. Neubauer, *The Yale Pharyngeal Residue Severity Rating Scale*, DOI 10.1007/978-3-319-29899-3_4,
© Springer International Publishing Switzerland 2016

binary (presence/absence) [4], (2) ordinal (to capture progressively increasing amounts) [1, 5–8], (3) estimation (amount of observed residue as an estimate of the percentage of the original bolus) [9–12], and (4) quantification (computer-based image analysis) [2, 13]. The sole purpose of all of these scales is to rate pharyngeal residue severity. These scales do not determine why residue occurs or ascertain the timing of residue occurrence during swallowing. No scale, to date, has provided in vivo, anatomically correct, image-based exemplars of graduated pharyngeal residue severity ratings against which clinicians can match their clinical judgments.

Fiberoptic endoscopic evaluation of swallowing (FEES) [14, 15] is a recognized, validated, and widely used technique to assess the pharyngeal phase of swallowing in order to diagnose dysphagia, recommend oral diets, and implement appropriate rehabilitation interventions, all with the goal of promoting safe and efficient swallowing [12, 16–19]. The endoscopist is alert to pre-swallow pooled secretions and post-swallow food residue in the pharynx. FEES has been shown to be more sensitive in identifying pharyngeal residue when compared to the videofluoroscopic swallow study (VFSS) [12, 19]. Since pharyngeal residue is an important predictor of swallowing success [1], it is important to ascertain residue severity in the valleculae and pyriform sinuses. However, to date, pharyngeal residue severity has not been described using an objective, anatomically correct, image-based, reliable, and validated rating scale based on FEES.

Standardized evaluation of depth of laryngeal penetration and aspiration has only been reported with the Penetration-Aspiration Scale (PAS) [20]. The PAS is an 8-point scale ranging from "1 (material does not enter the airway)" to "8 (material enters the airway, passes below the vocal folds, and no effort is made to eject)." The PAS was validated using VFSS and does not rate pharyngeal residue.

The presence of pre-swallow pooled secretions and post-swallow food residue in the *laryngeal vestibule* is an important sign of potential poor swallowing performance and increased aspiration risk later during FEES. Pooled secretions in the laryngeal vestibule were highly predictive of prandial aspiration in adults [1] and correlated with aspiration pneumonia in children [21]. However, determining bolus volume patterns in the laryngeal vestibule poses a particular problem as only trace and mild occur before caudal bolus flow results in aspiration. Therefore, the focus of the present study is solely on *pharyngeal residue.*

There is no objective, anatomically defined, image-based, reliable, and validated tool to rate severity of residue in the valleculae and pyriform sinuses during FEES. It would be advantageous for clinicians to be able to reliably determine, monitor, and share their patients' pharyngeal residue patterns. The purpose of this study was to develop, standardize, and validate the Yale Pharyngeal Residue Severity Rating Scale with the goal of providing objective, anatomically defined, image-based, reliable, and validated pharyngeal residue severity ratings based upon FEES.

Methods

Subjects

This study was approved by the Human Investigation Committee, Yale School of Medicine. Non-identified adult FEES evaluations performed at Yale-New Haven Hospital during 2013–2014 were used. Gender, age, ethnicity, and diagnosis were deemed not to influence the review of images by the raters.

Fiberoptic Endoscopic Evaluation of Swallowing (FEES)

The standard FEES protocol was followed with slight modifications [14, 15]. Briefly, each naris was examined visually and the scope passed through the most patent naris without administration of a topical anesthetic or vasoconstrictor to the nasal mucosa, thereby eliminating any potential adverse anesthetic reaction and assuring the endoscopist of a safe physiologic examination [22]. The base of the tongue, pharynx, and larynx were viewed, and swallowing was evaluated directly with six food boluses of approximately 5–10 cc volume each. Patients were encouraged to feed themselves, with assistance as needed, i.e., liquid with a straw or cup and puree with a spoon. All patients were allowed to swallow spontaneously, i.e., without a verbal command to swallow [23]. FEES equipment consisted of a distal chip flexible fiberoptic rhinolaryngoscope (KayPentax, Lincoln Park, NJ 07035, model VNL–117OK), light source (KayPentax, model EPK-1000), and a digital swallow workstation (KayPentax, model 7200).

The first food challenge consisted of three boluses of puree consistency (yellow pudding) followed by three thin liquid boluses (white, fat free, skim milk), as these colors have excellent contrast with pharyngeal and laryngeal mucosa [24]. A solid food challenge, i.e., graham cracker, was given only if the patient was dentate.

Severity Rating Definitions

Definitions were anatomically defined, were image based, and used a 5-point ordinal rating scale that encompassed the full range of severity ratings, i.e., none, trace, mild, moderate, and severe, for both the vallecula and pyriform sinus locations (Appendix).

Image Selection Process

In the absence of a criterion standard, two expert judges were considered the best referent standards. These two judges, with a combined 26 years of performing and interpreting FEES, reviewed a total of 261 FEES evaluations. All images were stored on a digital swallow workstation allowing for frame-by-frame editing. No audio cues were used. A total of 101 potential images were selected based on adequate image quality and severity criteria as defined in the Appendix. Consensus agreement allowed for selection of 25 potential final images, i.e., a no residue exemplar and three exemplars each of trace, mild, moderate, and severe vallecula and pyriform sinus residue. Hard-copy color images of the no residue, 12 vallecula, and 12 pyriform sinus images were randomized by residue location for hierarchical categorization by 20 raters.

Raters

A total of 20 raters from 18 different training institutions from around the world participated, i.e., otolaryngology residents ($n=11$), attending otolaryngologists ($n=5$), speech-language pathologists ($n=3$), and physician assistant ($n=1$). The raters had different durations of experience in performing and interpreting FEES evaluations (mean 8.3 years, range 2–27 years).

Raters were grouped by years of FEES experience and training status. Years of experience indicated that 10 raters had <4 years (mean 2.8 years, range 2–4 years) and 10 raters had > 5 years (mean 13.4 years, range 5–27 years). Training was done once, with random assignment of 10 raters to receive and 10 raters not to receive pre-rating training in determining vallecula and pyriform sinus pharyngeal residue severity ratings. Training included written definitions, visual depictions, verbal explanations, and clarifying questions/answers of the severity ratings. No training was limited to only written definitions and visual depictions of the severity ratings.

Reliability Testing

Intra-rater test-retest reliability, inter-rater reliability, and construct validity for severity ratings for all images were performed by the same two expert judges and 20 raters, 2 weeks apart, and with the order of image presentations randomized. This allowed for selection of the best representative exemplar in each severity rating, i.e., none, trace, mild, moderate, and severe.

Statistics

Analyses were done separately for vallecula and pyriform sinus locations. Therefore, there was a total of 260 ratings (20 raters rated 13 images) for each location at each time point. Kappa statistics and their standard errors were used to assess the extent of intra- and inter-rater reliability and construct validity [25]. *Intra-rater reliability* was calculated by pooling the 260 paired ratings and calculating a weighted kappa ([25], p. 223), weighted by the degree of disagreement, with comparison of the same image 2 weeks apart. A similar analysis was done to assess *construct validity* by comparing the initial ratings with the criterion standard ratings from the two expert judges. *Inter-rater reliability* was calculated using a multi-rater kappa ([25], p. 226) where the extent of agreement across raters was calculated for each of the five categories (none, trace, mild, moderate, and severe) followed by calculation of a weighted average of these category specific agreements, weighted by the number of ratings for each category. Weights were 1/13 for no residue and 3/13 for each of trace, mild, moderate, and severe residue. Kappa statistics +/– standard error (se) are reported. Kappa statistics were compared across subsets of years of experience and training using Z-statistics.

Results

Intra- and inter-rater reliability was 100 % for the two expert judges based on the rating of the 25 potential final scale images, i.e., a no residue exemplar and three examples each of trace, mild, moderate, and severe vallecula and pyriform sinus residue.

TABLE 4.1 Intra-rater test-retest reliability, inter-rater reliability, and construct validity kappa statistics (standard error) for vallecula and pyriform sinus residue ratings across all raters (n = 20)

Location[a]	Kappa (se)
Intra-rater reliability	
Vallecula	0.957(+0.014)
Pyriform sinus	0.854(+0.021)
Inter-rater reliability	
Vallecula	0.868(+0.011)
Pyriform sinus	0.751(+0.011)
Construct validity	
Vallecula	0.951(+0.014)
Pyriform sinus	0.908(+0.017)

[a]Total of 260 ratings for each location

The Yale Pharyngeal Residue Severity Rating Scale demonstrated excellent overall intra-rater kappa statistics for both locations, specifically (1) intra-rater reliability for vallecula (0.957 + 0.014) and pyriform sinus (0.854 + 0.021), (2) inter-rater reliability for vallecula (0.868 + 0.011) and pyriform sinus (0.751 + 0.011), and (3) construct validity for vallecula (0.951 + 0.014) and pyriform sinus (0.908 + 0.017) (Table 4.1).

Intra-rater kappa statistics were between 0.823 + 0.032 and 0.969 + 0.017 dependent upon the location of residue (vallecula or pyriform sinus) and raters' years of experience (Table 4.2). No differences by years of experience for intra-rater reliability for vallecula ($p = 0.38$) and pyriform sinus ($p = 0.17$) kappas were found. Inter-rater reliability for years of experience was not consistent, i.e., <4 years had higher kappas for vallecula ($p <0.001$) but lower kappas for pyriform sinus ($p <0.001$).

Intra-rater kappa statistics were between 0.838 + 0.033 and 0.989 + 0.008 dependent upon the location of residue (vallecula or pyriform sinus) and training versus no training (Table 4.3). A difference was found in favor of training with

TABLE 4.2 Intra-rater test-retest reliability and inter-rater reliability kappa statistics (standard error) for vallecula and pyriform sinus residue ratings based on years of experience ≤4 years ($n=10$) years versus ≥5 years ($n=10$)

Location[a]	Kappa (se)	Location	Kappa (se)
Intra-rater reliability			
Vallecula		Pyriform sinus	
≤4 years	0.968(+0.017)	≤4 years	0.823(+0.032)
≥5 years	0.946(+0.021)	≥5 years	0.881(+0.028)
$Z=0.82$		$Z=1.36$	
p value: 0.38		*p* value: 0.17	
Inter-rater reliability			
Vallecula		Pyriform sinus	
≤4 years	0.921(+0.022)	≤4 years	0.648(+0.022)
≥5 years	0.816(+0.022)	≥5 years	0.886(+0.022)
$Z=3.38$		$Z=7.68$	
p <0.001		*p* <0.001	

[a]Total of 130 ratings for each subset

higher vallecula kappas ($p=0.02$), but no difference was found for pyriform sinus kappas ($p=0.45$). Inter-rater kappa statistics were between $0.680+0.022$ and $0.961+0.022$ dependent upon the location of residue (vallecula or pyriform sinus) and training resulted in higher kappas for both locations ($p<0.001$).

Construct validity kappa statistics were between $0.848+0.031$ and 1.000 dependent upon the location of residue (vallecula or pyriform sinus) and either years of experience or training status (Table 4.4). More years of experience had higher kappa values for pyriform sinus ($p=0.001$), and there was no difference by years of experience for vallecula ($p=0.25$). Training again resulted in higher kappas for both vallecula ($p=0.007$) and pyriform sinus ($p=0.001$).

TABLE 4.3 Intra-rater test-retest reliability and inter-rater reliability kappa statistics (standard error) for vallecula and pyriform sinus residue based on training ($n=10$) versus no training ($n=10$)

Location[a]	Kappa (se)	Location	Kappa (se)
Intra-rater reliability			
Vallecula		Pyriform sinus	
Training	0.989(+0.008)	Training	0.838(+0.033)
No training	0.924(+0.026)	No training	0.870(+0.027)
$Z=2.39$		$Z=0.75$	
p value: 0.02		p value: 0.45	
Inter-rater reliability			
Vallecula		Pyriform sinus	
Training	0.961(+0.022)	Training	0.805(+0.022)
No training	0.777(+0.022)	No training	0.680(+0.022)
$Z=5.93$		$Z=4.03$	
$p<0.001$		$p<0.001$	

[a]Total of 130 ratings for each subset

Inter-rater reliability kappa statistics for re-randomized images rated 2 weeks later were between $0.670+0.022$ and $1.000+0.022$ for years of experience and between $0.698+0.022$ and $1.000+0.002$ for training (Table 4.5). More years of experience had higher kappa values for pyriform sinus ($p<0.001$), and there was no difference by years of experience for vallecula ($p=0.23$). Training did not result in higher kappa values for both vallecula ($p=0.21$) and pyriform sinus ($p=0.32$). Construct validity kappa statistics were between $0.870+0.027$ and 1.000 dependent upon the location of residue (vallecula or pyriform sinus) and either years of experience or training status. More years of experience did not result in higher kappa values for either vallecula ($p=0.20$) or pyriform sinus ($p=0.23$). Training did not result in higher kappa values for either vallecula ($p=0.17$) or pyriform sinus ($p=0.55$).

TABLE 4.4 Construct validity kappa statistics (standard error) for vallecula and pyriform sinus residue ratings based on years of experience and training

Location[a]	Kappa (se)	Location	Kappa (se)
Vallecula		Pyriform sinus	
Years of experience			
≤4 years	0.968(+0.017)	≤4 years	0.848(+0.031)
≥5 years	0.935(+0.023)	≥5 years	0.967(+0.013)
$Z = 1.15$		$Z = 3.54$	
p value: 0.25		p value: <0.001	
Training			
Training	0.989(+0.008)	Training	1.000(0.000)
No training	0.913(+0.027)	No training	0.881(+0.028)
$Z = 2.70$		$Z = 4.25$	
p value: 0.007		p value: <0.001	

The single image with the greatest inter-rater agreement for each residue severity level, i.e., none, trace, mild, moderate, and severe, and for each location, i.e., vallecula (Fig. 4.1) and pyriform sinus (Fig. 4.2) became the chosen exemplar for inclusion in the Yale Pharyngeal Residue Severity Rating Scale.

Discussion

The Yale Pharyngeal Residue Severity Rating Scale has achieved its stated goal of providing reliable and valid information regarding the location and severity of pharyngeal residue observed during FEES. Vallecula and pyriform sinus residue severity ratings (Figs. 4.1 and 4.2) showed overall excellent intra-rater reliability, inter-rater agreement, and construct validity. Importantly, repeat ratings 2 weeks later of the same but re-randomized images found that neither years of experience nor training status resulted in higher validity kappa values for vallecula and pyriform sinus ratings.

TABLE 4.5 Inter-rater reliability and construct validity kappa statistics (standard error) for re-randomized vallecula and pyriform sinus residue images rated 2 weeks later based on years of experience ≤4 ($n=10$) versus ≥5 years ($n=10$) and training ($n=10$) versus no training ($n=10$)

Location[a]	Kappa (se)	Location	Kappa (se)
Inter-rater reliability			
Vallecula		Pyriform sinus	
Inter-rater reliability			
Years of experience			
≤4 years	1.000(+0.022)	≤4 years	0.670(+0.022)
≥5 years	0.960(+0.022)	≥5 years	0.774(+0.022)
$Z=1.29$		$Z=3.35$	
p value: 0.23		*p* value: <0.001	
Training			
Training	1.000(+.022)	Training	0.698(+0.022)
No training	0.961(+0.022)	No training	0.726(+0.022)
$Z=1.26$		$Z=0.90$	
p value: 0.21		*p* value: 0.32	
Construct validity			
Vallecula		Pyriform sinus	
Years of experience			
≤4 years	1.000(0.000)	≤4 years	0.870(+0.027)
≥5 years	0.989(+0.008)	≥5 years	0.913(+0.024)
$Z=1.38$		$Z=1.19$	
p value: 0.20		*p* value: 0.23	
Training			
Training	1.000(0.000)	Training	0.881(+0.028)
No training	0.989(+0.008)	No training	0.903(+0.023)
$Z=1.38$		$Z=0.61$	
p value: 0.17		*p* value: 0.55	

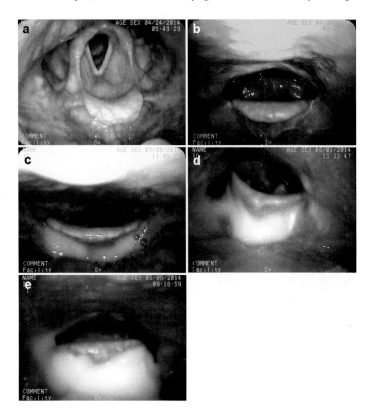

FIGURE 4.1 The vallecula images with the greatest inter-rater agreement for each residue level: (a) none, (b) trace, (c) mild, (d) moderate, and (e) severe

Therefore, proficiency in the use of the Yale Pharyngeal Residue Severity Rating Scale is readily achievable in a short period of time by clinicians from different specialty areas and with different levels of expertise.

The sole purpose of the Yale Pharyngeal Residue Severity Rating Scale is to allow clinicians and researchers rate post-swallow vallecula and pyriform sinus residue severity. Consistent with all other pharyngeal residue rating scales [1, 2, 4–13], the Yale Pharyngeal Residue Severity Rating Scale does not

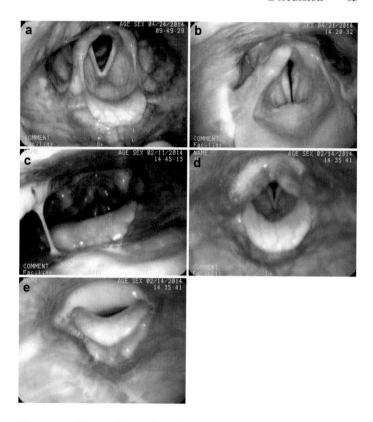

FIGURE 4.2 The pyriform sinus images with the greatest inter-rater agreement for each residue level: (**a**) none, (**b**) trace, (**c**) mild, (**d**) moderate, and (**e**) severe

determine why residue occurs or ascertain the timing of residue occurrence during swallowing. Since all patients have unique swallowing characteristics, it is up to the clinician to determine the why and when of residue occurrence during swallowing. The superiority of the Yale Pharyngeal Residue Severity Rating Scale is due to its anatomically defined and image-based construction resulting in excellent validity, easy administration and accurate interpretation by clinicians with a wide range of FEES experience, and generalizability to all individuals.

The utility, versatility, and efficacy of the Yale Pharyngeal Residue Severity Scale are easily demonstrated. For example, a representative pre-therapy swallow receives a severe vallecular residue severity rating (anatomically defined as the vallecula filled up to the epiglottic rim and with a corresponding image). An intervention strategy, such as effortful swallow or double swallow, is implemented for a set period of time, and a representative post-therapy swallow receives a mild vallecular residue severity rating (anatomically defined as mild pooling with epiglottic ligament visible and with a corresponding image). The clinician can now document efficacy of a specific treatment intervention and either stop, continue, or change strategies. Prior to the development and validation of the Yale Pharyngeal Residue Severity Rating Scale, objective documentation of therapeutic interventions was not possible.

The Yale Pharyngeal Residue Rating Scale works well for any swallow, whether it is the first, subsequent clearing, or last swallow. The clinician simply has to match their chosen swallow with its scale mate. In this way, it is possible to determine if spontaneous or volitional clearing swallows or a throat-clearing maneuver is actually helpful in reducing the amount of residue in the vallecula and pyriform sinuses. Since an important therapeutic goal is to aid pharyngeal clearing [1], this information can guide intervention strategies and promote safer swallowing. For example, it is now possible to determine objectively if drinking a small liquid bolus after a puree/solid bolus, an effortful swallow, a double swallow/bolus, a head turn to left or right, and a chin tuck are successful in reducing residue in the vallecula and pyriform sinus.

Since the anatomical definitions used by the Yale Pharyngeal Residue Scale are discrete, i.e., not continuous and image based, the severity rating is not affected by age, gender, or body habitus. For example, mild vallecula residue is defined as "epiglottic ligament visible." The shape and size of the vallecula are unimportant. As long as the lingual frenulum is visible, the severity rating is mild residue. This generalizability makes it possible to determine pharyngeal residue severity for any given individual.

The Yale Pharyngeal Residue Severity Rating Scale can be used for both clinical advantages and research opportunities. Clinically, clinicians can now accurately classify vallecula and pyriform sinus residue severity as none, trace, mild, moderate, or severe for diagnostic purposes, determination of functional therapeutic change, and precise dissemination of shared information. Future research uses include tracking outcome measures for clinical trials investigating various swallowing interventions, demonstrating efficacy of specific interventions to reduce pharyngeal residue, determining morbidity and mortality associated with pharyngeal residue severity in different patient populations, and improving the training and accuracy of FEES interpretation by students and clinicians.

Conclusions

The Yale Pharyngeal Residue Severity Rating Scale is a reliable, validated, anatomically defined, and image-based tool to determine residue location and severity based on FEES. Proficiency can be readily achieved with minimal training and at high levels of intra- and inter-rater reliability and construct validity. Clinical uses include, but are not limited to, accurate classification of vallecula and pyriform sinus residue severity patterns as none, trace, mild, moderate, or severe for diagnostic purposes, determination of functional therapeutic change, and precise dissemination of shared information. Scientific uses include, but are not limited to, tracking outcome measures, demonstrating efficacy of interventions to reduce pharyngeal residue, investigating morbidity and mortality in relation to pharyngeal residue severity, and improving training and accuracy of FEES interpretation by students and clinicians. The Yale Pharyngeal Residue Severity Rating Scale is an important addition to the deglutologist's toolbox and can be used with confidence for both clinical and research purposes.

Appendix

Definitions for severity of vallecula residue			
I	None	0 %	No residue
II	Trace	1–5 %	Trace coating of the mucosa
III	Mild	5–25 %	Epiglottic ligament visible
IV	Moderate	25–50 %	Epiglottic ligament covered
V	Severe	>50 %	Filled to epiglottic rim

Definitions for severity of pyriform sinus residue			
I	None	0 %	No residue
II	Trace	1–5 %	Trace coating of mucosa
III	Mild	5–25 %	Up wall to quarter full
IV	Moderate	25–50 %	Up wall to half full
V	Severe	>50 %	Filled to aryepiglottic fold

References

1. Murray J, Langmore SE, Ginsberg S, Dostie A. The significance of oropharyngeal secretions and swallowing frequency in predicting aspiration. Dysphagia. 1996;11:99–103.
2. Pearson WG, Molfenter SM, Smith ZM, Steele CM. Image-based measurement of post-swallow residue: the Normalized Residue Ratio Scale. Dysphagia. 2013;28:167–77.
3. Logemann J. Evaluation and treatment of swallowing disorders. 2nd ed. Austin: Pro-Ed; 1998.
4. Dejaeger E, Pelemans W, Ponette E, Joosten E. Mechanisms involved in postdeglutition retention in the elderly. Dysphagia. 1997;12:63–7.
5. Farneti D. Pooling score: an endoscopic model for evaluating severity of dysphagia. Acta Otorhinological Italica. 2008;28:135–40.
6. Tohara H, Nakane A, Murata S, Mikushi S, Ouchi Y, Wakasugi Y, Takashima M, Chiba Y, Uematsu H. Inter- and inter-rater reliability in fibroptic endoscopic evaluation of swallowing. J Oral Rehabil. 2010;37:884–91.

7. Kaneoka AS, Langmore SE, Krisciunas GP, Field K, Scheel R, McNally E, Walsh MJ, O'Dea MB, Cabral H. The Boston Residue and Clearance Scale: preliminary reliability and validity testing. Folia Phoniatr Logop. 2014;65:312–7.

8. Donzelli J, Brady S, Wesling M, Craney M. Predictive value of accumulated oropharyngeal secretions for aspiration during video nasal endoscopic evaluation of the swallow. Ann Otol Rhinol. 2003;112:469–75.

9. Han TR, Paik NJ, Park JW. Quantifying swallowing function after stroke: a functional dysphagia scale based on videofluoroscopic studies. Arch Phys Med Rehabil. 2001;82:677–82.

10. Eisenhuber E, Schima W, Schober E, Pokieser P, Stadler A, Scharitzer M, Oschatz E. Videofluoroscopic assessment of patients with dysphagia: pharyngeal retention is a predictive factor for aspiration. AJR Am J Roentgenol. 2002;178:393–8.

11. Logemann JA, Williams RB, Rademaker A, Pauloski BR, Lazarus CL, Cook I. The relationship between observations and measures of oral and pharyngeal residue from videofluorography and scintigraphy. Dysphagia. 2005;20:226–31.

12. Kelly AM, Leslie P, Beale T, Payten C, Drinnan MJ. Fibreoptic endoscopic evaluation of swallowing and videofluoroscopy: does examination type influence perception of pharyngeal severity? Clin Otolaryngol. 2006;31:425–32.

13. Dyer JC, Leslie P, Drinnan MJ. Objective computer-based assessment of valleculae residue: is it useful? Dysphagia. 2008;23:7–15.

14. Langmore SE, Schatz K, Olsen N. Fiberoptic endoscopic examination of swallowing safety: a new procedure. Dysphagia. 1988;2:216–9.

15. Leder SB, Murray JT. Fiberoptic endoscopic evaluation of swallowing. Phys Med Rehabil Clin No Am. 2008;19:787–801.

16. Wu CH, Hsiao TY, Chen JC, Yeun-Chung C, Shiann-Yann L. Evaluation of swallowing safety with fiberoptic endoscope: comparison with videofluoroscopic technique. Laryngoscope. 1997;107:396–401.

17. Leder SB, Sasaki CT, Burrell MI. Fiberoptic endoscopic evaluation of dysphagia to identify silent aspiration. Dysphagia. 1998;13:19–21.

18. Leder SB, Karas DE. Fiberoptic endoscopic evaluation of swallowing in the pediatric population. Laryngoscope. 2000;110:1132–6.

19. Kelly AM, Drinnan MJ, Leslie P. Assessing penetration and aspiration: how do videofluoroscopy and fiberoptic endoscopic evaluation of swallowing compare? Laryngoscope. 2007;117:1723–7.

20. Rosenbek JC, Robbins JA, Roecker EB, Coyle JC, Wood JL. A penetration-aspiration scale. Dysphagia. 1996;11:93–8.
21. Link DT, Willging JP, Miller CK, Cotton RT, Rudolph CD. Pediatric laryngoscopic sensory testing during flexible endoscopic evaluation of swallowing: feasible and correlative. Ann Otol Rhinol Laryngol. 2000;109:899–905.
22. Leder SB, Ross DA, Briskin KB, Sasaki CT. A prospective, double-blind, randomized study on the use of topical anesthetic, vasoconstrictor, and placebo during transnasal flexible fiberoptic endoscopy. J Speech Lang Hear Res. 1997;40:1352–7.
23. Daniels SK, Schroeder MF, DeGeorge PC, Corey D, Rosenbek JC. Effects of verbal cue on bolus flow during swallowing. J Am Speech Lang Pathol. 2007;16:140–7.
24. Leder SB, Acton LA, Lisitano HL, Murray JT. Fiberoptic endoscopic evaluation of swallowing (FEES) with and without blue dyed food. Dysphagia. 2005;20:157–62.
25. Fleiss JL. Statistical methods for rates and proportions. New York: Wiley; 1981.

Chapter 5
The Epiglottis: The Most Prominent Anatomical Structure in the Pharynx

Introduction

> The weight of evidence then is in favor of the view that the epiglottis is not essential to the deglutition of dogs and cats. We cannot of course assume from this alone that the epiglottis is equally inessential to deglutition in man. Walton, 1878, p. 307 [1]

Since the nineteenth century, the epiglottis, being the most prominent structure in the pharynx, has been the subject of scientific inquiry. While some scientists regarded the adult human epiglottis as vestigial with no important physiologic swallow function [1–6], others felt it played a key role in preventing deglutitive aspiration [7–11]. And so, the controversy continues.

While both historical and contemporary research reported that successful deglutition can occur when the epiglottis was impaired or even destroyed by either disease or surgery [1, 2, 5, 6, 12], others contended that the epiglottis was important for airway protection during deglutition by providing a protective valve-like action during swallowing [7] or that specific

Leder SB, Burrell MI, Van Daele DJ. Epiglottis is not essential for successful swallowing in humans. Ann Otol Rhinol Laryngol. 2010;119:795–8 (Used and modified permission from SAGE Journals).

movement patterns [8–10] or positions [11] were indicative of aspiration risk. However, the exact physiologic mechanisms that cause epiglottic downfolding have only been partially explained [4, 13].

More recent computer-based radiographic imaging analysis revealed that epiglottic downfolding during swallowing in adult man was comprised of two distinct processes [14]. The first epiglottic movement occurred at the attachment of the epiglottis to the thyroid cartilage and brings the epiglottis from its semi-vertical resting position to a horizontal orientation concurrently with elevation of the larynx and hyoid bone during swallowing. The second epiglottic movement occurred as the bolus passes through the larynx and brings the upper one-third of the epiglottis below the horizontal plane. Post-deglutitive descent of the larynx and hyoid bone allowed the epiglottis to return passively to its pre-swallow upright position.

The epiglottis is best developed and serves its most effective function in macrosmatic animals, e.g., deer, sheep, dogs, horses, rodents, and elephants, due to its high location in the pharynx permitting it to rest on the soft palate. This intra-narial position provides an important protective biological function by isolating the oral cavity from the remainder of the respiratory tract to allow for maintenance of olfaction for threat detection during feeding [5, 15]. In microsmatic animals, e.g., cats, monkeys, apes, sea-dwelling mammals, and adult man, the poorly developed epiglottis does not reach the nasopharynx. In man, maturational descent of the larynx occurs between 4 and 6 months of age and results in a change from obligate nasal breathing to oral tidal respiration [16]. Maturational descent also results in an unfilled gap between the epiglottis and the soft palate and a de facto increase in aspiration risk due to the lowered position of the larynx in the upper respiratory tract.

The purposes of the present study are to use a human model to confirm Walton's [1] findings of successful deglutition following isolated surgical epiglottectomy in the dog and cat models and to corroborate Howes' [2] assertion of the nonessential purpose of the human epiglottis to protectively valve the larynx to prevent deglutitive aspiration.

Methods

Using the adult human model, videofluoroscopic swallowing studies (VFSS) based on three cases with different etiologies for isolated epiglottectomy are presented. Only the epiglottis was removed, sparing the adjacent base of tongue, aryepiglottic folds, and pre-epiglottic space. This study was approved by the Human Investigation Committee, Yale University School of Medicine.

All VFSS were performed with each subject seated upright in the fluoroscopy chair and viewed in the lateral plane (Philips Medical Systems, Hamburg, Germany, Model SRO 33 100). The image included the lips anteriorly to the pharyngeal wall posteriorly and the soft palate superiorly to the sixth cervical vertebra inferiorly. All subjects were tested with all food consistencies, i.e., single-contrast barium and single-contrast barium thinned 50 % with water, puree + barium, and solid + barium (E-Z-Paque, E-Z-EM, Westbury, NY). Rapid sequence imaging at 3/s was used during swallowing of approximately 5–10 cc liquid bolus volumes.

Case #1: Traumatic Epiglottectomy with Rapid Swallowing Success

The patient is a 42-year-old male with a large, almost decapitation-type injury of his neck status post motor vehicle crash. Exploration of the neck wound allowed identification of the carotid arteries and jugular veins bilaterally. These were somehow spared injury, but the epiglottis was now disconnected from the thyroid cartilage and only minimally attached to the pharyngeal mucosa. There was a large laceration extending back posteriorly on the right side in the posterior

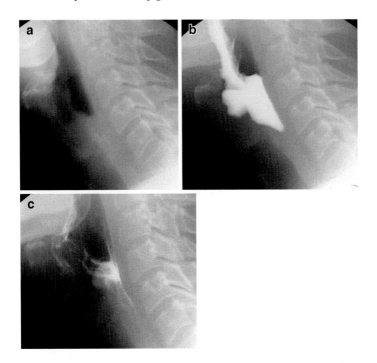

FIGURE 5.1 VFSS following traumatic epiglottectomy. No aspiration: (**a**) pre-swallow, (**b**) during the swallow, or (**c**) post-swallow

pharyngeal wall down to the prevertebral fascia. The laceration was carried out to the left side to the lateral pharyngeal wall. The epiglottis was removed and submitted to pathology. The posterior and lateral pharyngeal wall incisions were closed while maintaining meticulous hemostasis. The tongue base was then attached to the thyrohyoid membrane.

The patient was kept nil by mouth with nasogastric tube feeding for 22 days postoperatively to allow time for healing. A VFSS (Fig. 5.1a–c) indicated successful swallowing without aspiration with all food consistencies tested despite absence of an epiglottis, i.e., single-contrast barium and single-contrast barium thinned 50 % with water, puree + barium, and solid + barium. A small amount of pyriform sinus residue was cleared with a double swallow.

Case #2: Surgical Epiglottectomy with a Short-Term Period of Dysphagia due to Postoperative Edema Followed by Swallowing Success

The patient is a 51-year-old female with a diagnosis of squamous cell carcinoma of the supraglottis and is postoperative both supraglottic laryngectomy and external beam radiation therapy. The patient takes all nutrition orally, has not had an aspiration pneumonia, and has not lost weight postoperatively. She does complain of odynophagia.

A VFSS (Fig. 5.2a–c) performed 6 months postoperatively indicated successful swallowing without aspiration with all food consistencies tested despite absence of an epiglottis, i.e., single-contrast barium and single-contrast barium thinned 50 % with water, puree + barium, and solid + barium. The patient did not complain of odynophagia during testing. It was recommended she continue with her current nutrition regimen, i.e., regular consistency oral diet.

Case #3: Long-Term Adaptation to Cancerous Erosion of the Entire Epiglottis with Successful Swallowing Maintained

The patient is a 70-year-old female who presented with a large, exophytic mass that completely replaced her epiglottis. Biopsy revealed squamous cell carcinoma, and she was staged as having a T2NoMo (stage II) lesion of the epiglottis. She received a full course of external beam radiation therapy with concurrent chemotherapy. Posttreatment fiberoptic laryngoscopy revealed absence of an epiglottis with true vocal folds mobile bilaterally. The patient takes all nutrition orally, has not had an aspiration pneumonia, and has only lost approximately 4 lb 1 month post-chemoradiotherapy.

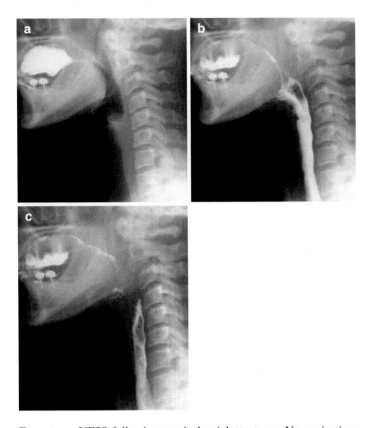

FIGURE 5.2 VFSS following surgical epiglottectomy. No aspiration: (**a**) pre-swallow, (**b**) during the swallow, or (**c**) post-swallow

A VFSS (Fig. 5.3a–c) performed 2 months post-chemoradiotherapy indicated successful swallowing without aspiration with all food consistencies tested despite absence of an epiglottis, i.e., single-contrast barium, puree + barium, and solid + barium. It was recommended she continue with her current nutrition regimen, i.e., regular consistency oral diet, and add high-calorie supplements to increase weight.

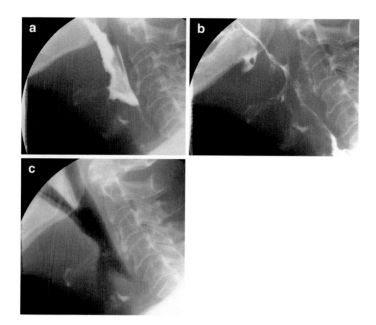

FIGURE 5.3 VFSS following cancerous erosion epiglottectomy. No aspiration: (**a**) pre-swallow, (**b**) during the swallow, or (**c**) post-swallow

Discussion

The present study found that successful swallowing with all food consistencies, i.e., thin liquid, puree, and solid, without aspiration occurred for all adult human participants following isolated epiglottectomy from three diverse etiologies: specifically, trauma with rapid swallowing success, surgical with a short-term period of dysphagia due to postoperative edema followed by swallowing success, and long-term adaptation to cancerous erosion of the entire epiglottis with successful swallowing maintained.

Although the epiglottis has been described as a key primary valve of airway protection during swallowing [7] and that specific epiglottic movement patterns [8–10] and positions [11] may be indicative of aspiration risk, the human case studies reported here support the converse view, i.e., the epiglottis is a nonessential [1, 2], vestigial [4], and degenerate [5] organ in man. In addition, since an epiglottis exhibits many different movement patterns and positions due to its passive role during swallowing [14], epiglottic movement does not appear to be a causative marker of aspiration risk.

It is important to note that all three patients presented with intact central and peripheral nervous systems. Deglutition is controlled by complex neuromotor functioning with a substantial component of biological redundancy that permits adaptation to, for example, altered anatomy [17]. In the presence of intact neuromuscular functioning, successful swallowing can occur following isolated epiglottectomy, but when neuromuscular damage is present, an intact epiglottis may perform a protective function during deglutition.

Most importantly, an epiglottis allows for formation of a vallecula on its lingual surface where small amounts of food may collect after the initial swallow [5]. With the epiglottis gone, e.g., due to trauma, surgery, or cancer, there is no longer a vallecula, and post-swallow residue may rest directly on the true vocal folds. However, as illustrated by the present human case studies, patients readily adapt to isolated epiglottectomy and avoid tracheal aspiration.

Conclusions

> The old belief in the valvular action of the human epiglottis is well-nigh exploded. We know from actual observation, little or nothing in support thereof, and it finds a resting-place among the phantasies born of a too exclusive contemplation on self. Howes, 1889, p. 267 [2]

Victorian era scientists, although lacking modern imaging technology, were keen observers and interpreters of the natural world. Their elucidations on the anatomy, physiology, and biological purposes of the role of the epiglottis in deglutition have proven to be correct. Although their work has been lost to the current generation of scientists, reading Walton [1] and

Howes [2] provides both historical perspective and valuable insight. Most importantly, their results have passed the true measure of scientific discovery—"the test of time."

References

1. Walton GL. The function of the epiglottis in deglutition and phonation. J Physiol. 1878;1:303–20.
2. Howes GB. Rabbit with an intra-narial epiglottis, with a suggestion concerning the phylogeny of the mammalian respiratory apparatus. J Anat Physiol. 1889;23:263–72.
3. Pressman J, Keleman G. Physiology of the larynx. Physiol Rev. 1955;35:506–54.
4. Zemlin WR. Speech and hearing science. 3rd ed. Englewood Cliffs: Prentice-Hall, Inc.; 1988.
5. Kirchner JA. Physiology of the larynx. 3rd ed. Washington, DC: American Academy of Otolaryngology–Head and Neck Surgery Foundation, Inc; 1986.
6. Medda BK, Kern M, Ren J, Xie P, Ulualp SO, Lang IM, et al. Relative contribution of various airway protective mechanisms to prevention of aspiration during swallowing. Am J Gastrointest Liver Physiol. 2003;284:G933–9.
7. Ardran GM, Kemp FH. The mechanism of the larynx. Br J Radiol. 1967;40:372–89.
8. Perlman AL, Grayhack JP, Booth BM. The relationship of vallecular residue to oral involvement, reduced hyoid elevation, and epiglottic function. J Speech Hear Res. 1992;35:734–41.
9. Perlman AL, Booth BM, Grayhack JP. Videofluoroscopic predictors of aspiration in patients with oropharyngeal dysphagia. Dysphagia. 1994;9:90–5.
10. Garon BR, Huang Z, Hommeyer S, Eckmann D, Stern GA, Ormiston C. Epiglottic dysfunction: abnormal epiglottic movement patterns. Dysphagia. 2002;17:57–68.
11. Mong A, Levine MS, Rubesin SE, Laufer I. Epiglottic carcinoma as a cause of laryngeal penetration and aspiration. Am J Radiol. 2003;180:207–11.
12. Zeitels SM, Vaughan CW, Domanowski GF, Fuleihan NS, Simpson GT. Laser epiglottectomy: endoscopic technique and indications. Otolaryngol Head Neck Surg. 1990;103:337–43.
13. Ekberg O, Sigurjonsson S. Movement of the epiglottis during deglutition: a cineradiographic study. Gastrointest Rad. 1982;7:101–7.

14. Vandaele DJ, Perlman AL, Cassell MD. Intrinsic fibre architecture and attachments of the human epiglottis and their contributions to the mechanism of deglutition. J Anat. 1995;186:1–15.
15. Negus VE. The comparative anatomy and physiology of the larynx. London: W. Heinemann Medical Books; 1949.
16. Sasaki CT, Levine PA, Laitman JT, Crelin ES. Postnatal descent of the epiglottis in man. Arch Otolaryngol. 1977;103:169–71.
17. Logemann JA. Evaluation and treatment of swallowing disorders. 2nd ed. Austin: Pro-Ed; 1998.

Chapter 6
Really, How Easy Is It to Use the Yale Pharyngeal Residue Severity Rating Scale?

Introduction

The Yale Pharyngeal Residue Severity Rating Scale, being anatomically defined and image based, has demonstrated excellent intra-rater agreement, inter-rater reliability, and construct validity regardless of raters' medical specialty, years of FEES experience, or prior training in the use of the scale [1]. The health-care professionals included the specialty areas of speech-language pathology and otolaryngology, years of experience spanned 2–10 years, and training included didactic instruction on use of the scale. These clinician raters, however, all had medical backgrounds and a working knowledge of FEES.

We have stated that the Yale Pharyngeal Residue Severity Rating Scale is easy to use and excellent results are readily achievable with a minimal amount of prior use. Corroboration of these claims by raters with absolutely no training in use of the scale, no medical background, and no experience with FEES is, therefore, of interest. The purpose of this study was to determine if totally naïve raters with absolutely no training in use of the scale, no medical training, and no FEES experience were able to correctly hierarchically categorize the four final images of trace, mild, moderate, and severe vallecula and pyriform sinus residue severity rating patterns which comprise the Yale Pharyngeal Residue Severity Rating Scale [1].

S.B. Leder, P.D. Neubauer, *The Yale Pharyngeal Residue Severity Rating Scale*, DOI 10.1007/978-3-319-29899-3_6, © Springer International Publishing Switzerland 2016

Methods

Subjects

A total of ten participants with no medical training and no experience in either performing or interpreting FEES evaluations participated. Professions included were administrative assistants ($n=8$), environmental services ($n=1$), and law enforcement ($n=1$). Table 6.1 shows participant demographics.

Procedures

No training in use of the scale was given. The naïve raters were presented with randomly shuffled hard-copy images of the four vallecula and four pyriform sinus severity residue patterns from the Yale Pharyngeal Residue Severity Rating Scale, i.e., trace, mild, moderate, and severe, and instructed to organize them hierarchically from least amount of residue to most amount of residue. The images were then assigned a rating number, with 1 representing trace, 2 representing mild, 3 representing moderate, and 4 representing severe residue, i.e., 4 answers per rater or 4×10 raters = 40 answers. Agreement was evaluated between the hierarchical categorization from the naïve raters and the images from the Yale Pharyngeal Residue Severity Rating Scale.

TABLE 6.1 Participant demographics

Gender	Age (years)	Profession
2 males	Age range: 24–55 years	Environmental services ($n=1$)
		Law enforcement ($n=1$)
8 females	Age range: 22–65 years	Administrative assistants ($n=8$)

Results

All ten raters were able to correctly hierarchically categorize the pharyngeal severity ratings for both vallecular and pyriform sinus locations. Specifically, there was 100 % correct categorization for the 10 naïve raters for vallecula severity ratings and 90 % for pyriform sinus ratings when compared with the images from the Yale Pharyngeal Residue Severity Rating Scale.

Discussion

The Yale Pharyngeal Residue Severity Rating Scale has been shown to be intuitively easy to use and with a high degree of accuracy. Even naïve raters with absolutely no medical background and no experience performing or interpreting FEES evaluations were nonetheless able to correctly hierarchically rate images of vallecula and pyriform sinus residue patterns into trace, mild, moderate, and severe categories with a very high degree of accuracy, i.e., 90–100 %, respectively.

Conclusions

These findings both corroborate and add to the overall clinical robustness of the Yale Pharyngeal Residue Severity Rating Scale and support its use by clinicians from all medical and even nonmedical (!) specialties, regardless of background experience, training in use of the scale, or years of experience performing and interpreting FEES.

Reference

1. Neubauer PD, Rademaker AW, Leder SB. The Yale pharyngeal residue severity rating scale: an anatomically defined and image-based tool. Dysphagia. 2015;30:521–8. doi:10.1007/s00455-015-9631-4.

Chapter 7
Final Thoughts

Ever since its publication, we have been using and incorporating the Yale Pharyngeal Residue Severity Rating Scale [1] into our daily clinical care of patients. The scale's positive attributes are summarized in Table 7.1. The use of the scale makes it easy to observe and rate vallecula and pyriform sinus residue severity during fiberoptic endoscopic evaluation of swallowing (FEES). From a clinical perspective, many patients exhibit moderate or even severe residue patterns on the initial bolus swallow, but then the residue will diminish or clear and be recategorized as mild, trace, or even no residue remaining due to the clearing effects of the subsequent swallow. The endoscopist should report these positive changes for a number of reasons.

First, a spontaneous second (or even third) clearing swallow is a positive predictor of airway protection and decreased aspiration risk [2]. Second, from a therapeutic perspective, the patient can and should be instructed to perform a second volitional swallow with the goal of clearing post-swallow pharyngeal residue. The Yale Pharyngeal Residue Severity Rating Scale provides the treating clinician with objective documentation of the success of this therapeutic intervention. Third, from a research perspective, different strategies to promote a successful swallow can be trialed, e.g., double-swallow, swallow-clear throat-swallow again, and effortful swallow, all with the goal of clearing excess vallecula and pyriform sinus residue and thereby decreasing potential aspiration risk.

S.B. Leder, P.D. Neubauer, *The Yale Pharyngeal Residue Severity Rating Scale*, DOI 10.1007/978-3-319-29899-3_7,
© Springer International Publishing Switzerland 2016

TABLE 7.1 Summary of the advantages provided by the Yale Pharyngeal Residue Severity

1. Provides reliable, valid, and generalizable information regarding the location (vallecula and pyriform sinus) and severity (none, trace, mild, moderate, or severe) of pharyngeal residue during FEES

2. Is the only anatomically defined and image-based tool to determine vallecula and pyriform sinus residue severity

3. Works with any swallow: first, subsequent clearing

4. Is easy to use without a steep learning curve by both inexperienced and experienced endoscopists

5. Diagnostic uses include determination of vallecula and pyriform sinus residue severity, documentation of functional change during testing, and precise dissemination of shared information

6. Clinical uses include accurate classification of vallecula and pyriform sinus residue severity patterns as none, trace, mild, moderate, and severe in order to track success of therapeutic interventions

7. Research and scientific uses include tracking outcome measures, demonstrating efficacy of specific interventions to reduce pharyngeal residue, investigating morbidity and mortality in relation to pharyngeal residue severity patterns, and improving training and accuracy of FEES interpretation by students and clinicians

Two of the most important advantages of using the Yale Pharyngeal Residue Severity Rating Scale are the abilities to track changes due to swallow therapy over time and share reliable and validated judgments of vallecula and pyriform sinus residue severity patterns with fellow clinicians who are in the same institution or from around the world. In this current health-care environment where payment for care is predicated upon demonstration of positive therapeutic interventions and functional changes in health-care outcomes, it behooves all clinicians to determine if their interventions can be analyzed in an objective manner and can be repeatable by other clinicians. With regard to determining pharyngeal residue severity and success in its reduction, using the Yale Pharyngeal Residue Severity Rating Scale allows you, as the treating clinician, to use this tool in a valid, reliable, and generalizable manner to justify your hard work and document your patient's progress. Positive outcomes data are the only way to get reimbursed for services from the insurance companies and other funding agencies.

Similarly, in this mobile society, patients may seek out diagnostics at one institution and therapy at another. This certainly is the case in the acute care setting where ever decreasing lengths of stay which lead to rapid transit to rehabilitation facilities is now the norm [3]. The use of the Yale Pharyngeal Residue Severity Rating Scale allows for seamless and continuous tracking of progress in a longitudinal manner as the patient improves, for example, after a stroke, traumatic brain injury, or treatment for head and neck cancer. In this way, appropriate continuity of care and therapeutic changes can be documented to guide future therapy and justify reimbursement of services.

We trust that the information provided in our book will be the foundation on which to both base your confidence and document clinical improvement when you use the Yale Pharyngeal Residue Severity Rating Scale with your patients. We developed and validated the Yale Pharyngeal Residue Severity Rating Scale based on FEES for your use in order to promote optimal patient care. We firmly believe that the Yale Pharyngeal Residue Severity Rating Scale is a valuable addition to be incorporated into the deglutologist's toolbox for everyday use for both diagnostic and therapeutic purposes in patients with pharyngeal phase dysphagia.

The Yale Pharyngeal Residue Severity Rating Scale has changed our thinking and, therefore, our approach to identification, documentation, and intervention regarding vallecula and pyriform sinus residue severity. Importantly, it has enabled us to deliver both evidence-based and state-of-the-art clinical care to our patients. After all, when all is said and done, this is the ultimate clinical goal. We thank you for your open-mindedness and embrace of the Yale Pharyngeal Residue Severity Rating Scale into your daily clinical practice.

Best,
Steven B. Leder
Paul D. Neubauer

References

1. Neubauer PD, Rademaker AW, Leder SB. The Yale pharyngeal residue severity rating scale: an anatomically defined and image-based tool. Dysphagia. 2015;30:521–8.
2. Murray J, Langmore SE, Ginsberg S, Dostie A. The significance of oropharyngeal secretions and swallowing frequency in predicting aspiration. Dysphagia. 1996;11:99–103.
3. Leder SB, Suiter DM, Warner HL, Kaplan LJ. Initiating safe oral feeding in critically ill intensive care and step-down unit patients based on passing a 3-ounce (90 milliliters) water swallow challenge. J Trauma. 2011;70:1203–7.

Chapter 8
Images and Definitions
for Convenient Clinical Use

Electronic supplementary material The online version of this chapter
(doi:10.1007/978-3-319-29899-3_8) contains supplementary material,
which is available at http://link.springer.com/book/10.1007/978-3-319-29899-3.

S.B. Leder, P.D. Neubauer, *The Yale Pharyngeal Residue*
Severity Rating Scale, DOI 10.1007/978-3-319-29899-3_8,
© Springer International Publishing Switzerland 2016

Definitions for severity of vallecula residue.

I	None	0 %	No residue
II	Trace	1–5 %	Trace coating of the mucosa
III	Mild	5–25 %	Epiglottic ligament visible
IV	Moderate	25–50 %	Epiglottic ligament covered
V	Severe	>50 %	Filled to epiglottic rim

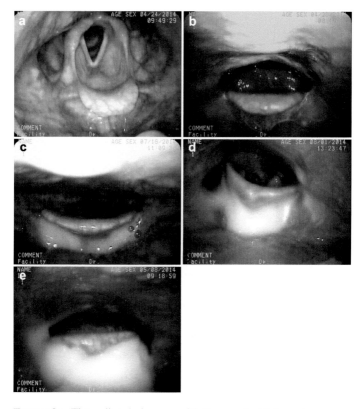

FIGURE 8.1 The vallecula images with the greatest inter-rater agreement for each residue level: (**a**) none, (**b**) trace, (**c**) mild, (**d**) moderate, and (**e**) severe

Definitions for severity of pyriform sinus residue.

I	None	0 %	No residue
II	Trace	1–5 %	Trace coating of mucosa
III	Mild	5–25 %	Up wall to quarter full
IV	Moderate	25–50 %	Up wall to half full
V	Severe	>50 %	Filled to aryepiglottic fold

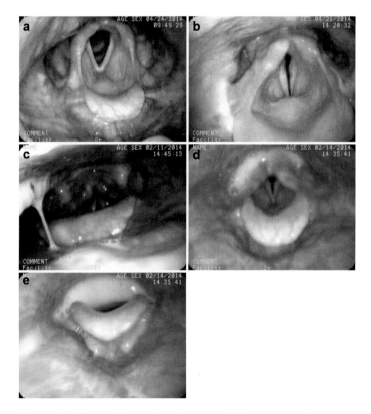

FIGURE 8.2 The pyriform sinus images with the greatest inter-rater agreement for each residue level: (**a**) none, (**b**) trace, (**c**) mild, (**d**) moderate, and (**e**) severe

Index

S.B. Leder, P.D. Neubauer, *The Yale Pharyngeal Residue
Severity Rating Scale*, DOI 10.1007/978-3-319-29899-3,
© Springer International Publishing Switzerland 2016

Printed in the United States
By Bookmasters